"Men and women in love should use their physical lovemaking to express their emotional love for one another."

In many societies and cultures all over the world, girls are *taught* from puberty how to sexually please their men. They learn the secret of really exquisite lovemaking and really true loving. They accept the whole of their bodies—hands, mouths, tongues, vaginas—as natural implements of lovemaking. They withhold none of their sexual talents because of a desire to be thought ladylike, a fear of being degraded, of behaving immorally. They are free of false feminine modesty, of feelings of guilt and shame, and of the myth that sex is mainly for men.

Other Titles by Robert Chartham in SIGNET Editions

☐ **ADVICE TO MEN.** The internationally famous sexologist and author of the bestselling **The Sensuous Couple** answers the most common and pressing sexual problems which trouble thousands of men.
(#Q5075—95¢)

☐ **SEX FOR ADVANCED LOVERS.** A sophisticated and most explicit manual for adults—a variety of techniques to enrich the pleasure of sexual love and overcome inhibitions. The author is an authority in the field of sex education.
(#T4429—75¢)

☐ **MAINLY FOR WIVES: The Art of Sex for Women.** An outspoken guide to the sex techniques that every woman should know to achieve a satisfying and mutually happy marriage. (#Q4884—95¢)

☐ **HUSBAND AND LOVER: The Art of Sex for Men.** A frank, authoritative guide describing in clear, everyday language the sex techniques every man should know in order to achieve a happy and satisfying marriage. (#Q4730—95¢)

THE NEW AMERICAN LIBRARY, INC.,
P.O. Box 999, Bergenfield, New Jersey 07621

Please send me the SIGNET BOOKS I have checked above. I am enclosing $_____ (check or money order—no currency or C.O.D.'s). Please include the list price plus 15¢ a copy to cover handling and mailing costs. (Prices and numbers are subject to change without notice.)

Name_____

Address_____

City_____State_____Zip Code_____
Allow at least 3 weeks for delivery

Advice to Women

by Robert Chartham, Ph.D.

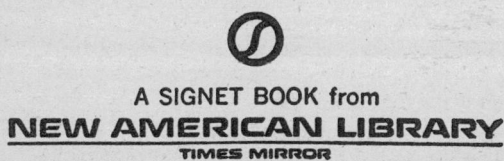

A SIGNET BOOK from
NEW AMERICAN LIBRARY
TIMES MIRROR

Copyright © 1971 by Robert Chartham

All rights reserved

Published by arrangement with the author

THIRD PRINTING

 SIGNET TRADEMARK REG. U.S. PAT. OFF. AND FOREIGN COUNTRIES
REGISTERED TRADEMARK—MARCA REGISTRADA
HECHO EN CHICAGO, U.S.A.

SIGNET, SIGNET CLASSICS, SIGNETTE, MENTOR AND PLUME BOOKS
are published by The New American Library, Inc.,
1301 Avenue of the Americas, New York 10019

FIRST PRINTING, APRIL, 1972

PRINTED IN THE UNITED STATES OF AMERICA

CONTENTS

		PAGE
	Introduction	7
1	Masturbation	15
2	Frigidity and Pseudo-frigidity	29
3	"My Husband Doesn't Know How to Rouse Me!"	40
4	"Is My Husband a Pervert?"	47
5	What is Sexual Excess?	62
6	The Lazy Husband	71
7	"My Husband Always Wants to Talk About Sex"	83
8	Being the Active Partner	94
9	"My Husband Has Been Unfaithful"	102
10	"My Husband Has Problems"	115

Introduction

Despite the fact that their normal experience of sex is much more simple and direct than a woman's, men's sexual problems tend to be more numerous and their causes more varied. They worry sincerely about the size and color of their penis, they get controversial about the advantages and disadvantages of circumcision, they are perturbed if their penis is bent or curved, depressed if their semen dribbles from the penis tip rather than spurts, they become inconsolable if they come too soon or have difficulty in coming at all, and they almost go out of their minds if something happens which makes them unable to obtain and/or sustain an erection, which prevents them from fulfilling their main role in life—the virile lover.

Apart from the most common of women's sexual problems—pseudo-frigidity, delayed orgasm, and occasional painful intercourse—the majority of women's sexual problems are nonetheless real for that, and they do affect very considerably the woman's enjoyment of sex, and they can color, and often tarnish, the whole sexual relationship. For the most part, they derive from criticism of the partner—his attitude toward and his much freer sexual behavior, his failure as a lover, his infidelity, his various -isms, and so on. Though, of course, very often the criticisms are valid, more often still they result from ignorance of both the man's and her own sexual roles combined with false modesty which has no place in the bed, or the bedroom, the bathroom or the bath, on the living-room couch or the hearthrug, or wherever else the lovemaking scene may be. With the exception of pseudo-frigidity, which is, in effect the woman's equivalent of the man's too rapid ejaculation and partial impotence, none of the woman's sexual problems need exist. I do not think they would exist if only she would make up her mind what her sexual role is.

I have set out my views on what her sexual role should

be in my book *Mainly For Wives*, and in every other place where I have written about women and physical sex. The days are past, I said and still say, when the woman could lie on her back and let things happen. Women are equal partners in lovemaking, I declared and still declare, but if they are equal partners, they must also accept equal responsibilities for seeing that their men receive as much satisfaction as they give.

What is the object of physical lovemaking, apart from procreation? Clearly one of its chief objects is to relieve the physical tensions which sexual arousal, in response to our sex drive, builds up in us from time to time. But most important of all, in my view, is the use we make of the acts we perform together to bring about this relief. Merely to respond physically to our sex urge is to indulge in what is described by that good old-fashioned word, not much heard nowadays—lust. To make love from lust is a contradiction in terms. It is the way animals mate—indiscriminately, without a thought for the partner, without any reasoning but by instinct. But because we humans are thinking creatures, capable of reasoning, we are also subject to emotions, and the strongest emotion we are capable of is love. Some of the other emotions, hate, for example, can be expressed in such ways that there can be no mistaking that it exists. Love, on the other hand, is much more difficult, because there are various categories of it—love for the marriage partner, love for parents and siblings, love for home—and because many of the ways in which we try to express it are also ways in which we try to express affection, i.e., love without a sexual content, we need something, some special expression to put our emotion across. It is not enough for a wife to attend to her husband's creature comforts, to mother his children, to greet him with kiss and embrace, nor is it enough for a husband to protect his wife, see that she wants for nothing that he can supply, to be her affectionate companion. They are ways of expressing love, but they do not express the closeness of spirit which emotional love involves. So how can we express our emotional love; how can we express in a way that the partner cannot misunderstand the oneness of minds and hearts which the couple truly in love represents?

Fortunately, there is a way. When the man puts his penis into his partner's vagina and buries it deep in her body, reaching toward her heart with it, as though he would pierce it, the two bodies become joined as they can become joined in no other way; and in no other way can they so closely represent with their bodies the union of their minds in love.

Because of this, I believe *that men and women in love should use their physical lovemaking to express their emotional love for one another.*

There is much more to lovemaking than the man putting his penis in the partner's vagina and swinging it backwards and forwards until he comes—and, if she is devilish lucky, until she comes, too. I am quite certain in my own mind that Nature intended physical lovemaking to be used as the expression of emotional love, because why else did she establish between men and women what I call the "arousal-gap"? It is a fact of life that the women who respond to orgasm solely by the friction of the vagina by the penis are so very rare that it is absolutely impossible to compute what fraction of the whole they are.

If the average man stimulates his penis directly, either by the vagina or some other means, from the very first second that his penis becomes erect he can bring himself to orgasm in from two to five minutes. The average woman, on the other hand, requires at least ten minutes, and more often than not fifteen minutes, or direct stimulation of the clitoral area to bring her to the point when another few seconds will bring her to orgasm. This is the "arousal-gap," and because of it, and because the natural end of lovemaking is that both should come while the penis is swinging in the vagina, foreplay (or love play, as it is also called) was invented. (Never was Necessity so much the Mother of Invention!)

And it is in foreplay that the very essence of lovemaking lies!

The clitoris is not the only sexually sensitive female zone. The nape of the neck, behind her ears, her throat and shoulders, her breasts and especially the nipples, her navel, her thighs and particularly her inner thighs, behind her knees, her perineum—the ridge between the lower edge of her vagina and her anus—her buttocks, and the full length of her spine, will all contribute to her sexual arousal if they are properly caressed by her partner.

So it is with the man. Though his penis, and especially the tip and the frenum—the little band of skin on the underside which joins the skin of the shaft to the membrane covering the penis head—is his most sensitive zone, he is also sensitive in the nape of his neck, behind his ears, his shoulders, his navel, his scrotum, his thighs and particularly his inner thighs, his perineum, his buttocks and the whole length of his spine respond with sexual arousal to the caresses of his partner.

The orgasm, i.e., the sensations that flush and flood through the body at the climax of lovemaking, gives greater relief to the physical tensions which the arousal builds up the more intense it is. The intensity of the orgasm is not always the same even in one individual. Many factors cause this differing intensity in the individual—the tiredness, the psychological mood, the circumstances and the surroundings in which love is made, are some of these factors.

But there is one factor which has a major effect on the intensity of all orgasms, and that is the skill with which the partners conduct the foreplay. In order to obtain a really intense orgasm on most occasions, there should be a series of near-climaxes, for both partners. That is to say, both should be brought to the threshold of the point-of-no-return several times. (The point-of-no-return is that point at which the involuntary muscles surrounding the root of the penis and the prostate muscle in the man, and the muscles surrounding the womb and the vagina which come into play at orgasm, at a certain moment of arousal begin to contract and relax and nothing the man or woman can do can stop them.) Then should there be a pause in the caresses until the sensations have died away; then stimulation should begin again and build up the sensations to the threshold of the point-of-no-return once more.

It is my view that the woman should be stimulated to this point four times before the partner puts his penis into her vagina for penis-vagina orgasm. Most women mount more rapidly to the threshold of the point-of-no-return once they have been brought there. The woman who needs ten minutes' stimulation to bring her on to this point the first time, reaches the point again in roughly six minutes, the third time in four minutes, and the fourth time in three minutes—provided her partner is an expert lover. If there is a pause of two minutes between each session of stimulation, then the minimum period of foreplay for her is 29 (say 30) minutes. In this time, the man will be brought to the point-of-no-return some seven or eight times. These sequences of stimulation will provide really intense orgasms for both partners.

To fill a minimum of 30 minutes a variety of caresses in the various sensitive zones is necessary if the whole operation is not to become a crashing bore. Men who are good and thoughtful lovers realize this; too many women do not. Or if they do, they find all sorts of excuses not to cooperate with their lovers, either in stimulating him, or in allowing themselves to be stimulated. It is, therefore, in this foreplay period that the opportunity is given to both partners to express through the skill of their arousal techniques how much they love the other. This is why I say that at every session of lovemaking both should, by their loveplay, try to induce in the partner the most voluptuous mounting arousal sensations that will lead to the most intense orgasms possible, taking mood and circumstances into account. This is also why I say that it is not enough for the woman merely to lie on her back and let things happen to her.

This passive giving, though I know she believes that she is expressing her love for her partner by merely letting him use her—and so she is, up to a point—does more than prevent her from expressing the true extent of her love. It also serves to prevent her from developing her lovemaking into the *equal* partnership, which I insist it should be.

If a woman can provide her partner with sensations that make his experience of lovemaking so much richer, how can she claim to be expressing her love for him if she withholds these caresses? Nor can she really expect him to use his lovemaking with her to express the real extent of his love for her. If only women would accept the principle of equal responsibilities in lovemaking, then half their sexual problems would never exist.

The time is past when the majority of women should make a reappraisal of their attitudes and approach to their own sexual behavior and the sexual behavior of their partners. I have to confess that I am confused by Women's Lib. It seems to me that at the same time that these women are demanding equality of status and opportunity, they are completely unaware of the fact that they already have equality of opportunity which, if they used it, would give them equality of status with men, at least in the love-bed. Furthermore, they do not seem to realize that equality of opportunity and status does carry with it equal responsibilities. Let them show that they are prepared to accept equal responsibilities and no one would be happier than men. This applies to practically every sphere of the male-female relationship in our society; it applies with special force to the sexual relationship.

I know that women are still emerging from the influence of the Victorians; that they are held back from being shameless hussies by such hang-ups as feminine modesty, fear of appearing unladylike in their bedroom behavior—who says this is a classless society?—fear of being degraded if you do certain things or permit certain things to be done to you, fear of being depraved for similar reasons. But for heaven's sake, if you believe your partner loves you—and I don't think you would be in bed with him if you didn't believe that—do you really think he will rate you as immodest, unladylike, or depraved, and will require you to do anything that will degrade you? Loving you as he does, he is trying to do just the opposite. Having set you on the throne of love, he is paying you the highest tribute he can with his offering to you of his body and all his lover's skills. Why can't you be gracious and show your appreciation by trying to reciprocate rather than just accepting all he offers you?

"And how," I can hear some of you saying, "are our partners going to react if we deprive them of their manly role of sexual aggressor?"

Man as natural sexual aggressor is a myth which has been foisted on succeeding generations by the fact that the woman has usurped for herself the role of victim in the name of femininity—whatever that is. Man has been forced to become the aggressor in sex, is today the aggressor in sex, only because if he doesn't come after it, he will never get it!

Aristophanes, the ancient Greek master of comedy-writing, began it, and Eric Linklater perpetuated it—the Lysistrata legend, I mean, the story of wives withholding themselves sexually from their warring husbands to persuade them to make peace. There is no historical equivalent, and I would not mind wagering that if any community of women withheld themselves from their menfolk they would quickly regret it. Poor substitute though it may be by the reckoning of heterosexuals, men can and do quickly compensate for the loss of conjugal rights. Look what happens in boys' schools, armies, navies, air forces, and prisons. Either the boy or the man contents himself with auto-sex, or seeks a deeper consolation in homo-sex.

Women, don't you understand that *you* hold the secret of truly successful and satisfying lovemaking? Do you realize that even the most fantastic lover in the world, though he may provide a really rich experience for you, is deprived of a similar experience by you if you will not also be his lover?

You probably haven't heard, as I have, men who have made love to women who have made love to them in return, express their amazed but heady appreciation of the loving of these women, women who have emerged from the dark undergrowth of femininity into the sunlight of sexual realization. No paeans in praise of victories in war have resounded with so much gratitude.

In many societies and cultures all over the world which we dismiss as inferior to our own, girls are *taught* from puberty how sexually to please their men. How can you be superior, if you are inferior to them as lovers?

I repeat, you women hold the secret of really successful lovemaking and really true loving. You have hands, mouths, tongues, and vaginas! For pity's sake, use them! But to get the best out of them, you have to accept them, indeed you have to accept the whole of your bodies, as natural implements of lovemaking. You must withhold none of your sexual talents because of a desire to be thought ladylike, a fear of being degraded, of behaving immorally. You must free yourself of your feminine modesty, of your feelings of guilt or shame, and of your belief that sex is mainly for men. If you can do that, then the great majority of your problems will cease to exist.

Chapter ONE

Masturbation

Masturbation means stimulating any of the sensitive zones of the body in order to obtain sexual arousal and orgasm by any means other than by the movement of the penis in the vagina. Usually it refers to self-stimulation in private or to stimulation by a member of the same sex (when it is known as mutual masturbation). If a man and a woman stimulate each other to orgasm without penis-vagina contact, it is called "heavy petting"; if, however, such stimulation is used as a preliminary to full intercourse, i.e., intercourse that ends with the penis in the vagina, it is called foreplay or loveplay.

When a man masturbates, he usually takes hold of his erect penis in his hand, or the head of the penis between two fingers and a thumb, and rubs it up and down until the very sensitive nerves in the penis head produce an orgasm. When a woman masturbates, she usually rubs her clitoris with her finger until she comes. There are, however, many ways in which both sexes can masturbate themselves. For example, quite a large number of men masturbate by lying on their stomachs, and by thrusting with their buttocks as they would do if the penis were in the vagina, they rub their penis against whatever they are lying on until they come. Besides finger-manipulation of the clitoris, one of the most common female ways of masturbating is by pressing the thighs very tightly together until the climax arrives. A few men and women are so sexually sensitive that they can bring themselves to orgasm by stimulation of the nipples only.

In the introductory chapter I referred to the difference there is between men and women in their respective speeds in responding to sexual arousal and climax; the average man takes between two and five minutes, the average woman ten to fifteen minutes. This difference is also reflected in the male and female experience of orgasm. When a man comes, the sensations are concentrated in his penis, scrotum, loins, lower belly, and upper thighs; in other words, he feels the voluptuous flushings in the concentrated area of his genitals and their immediate surroundings. When the woman comes, however, though she experiences the greater intensity of sensations in her genital area, ripples of sensation spread through her until practically the whole of her body is flushed with voluptuousness.

In its turn, this difference in experience is reflected in the man's and woman's experience of actual arousal. As soon as he is the slightest bit aroused his penis begins to swell and as the arousal becomes more marked, so the penis grows until it is completely changed from the limp, modest-appearing, almost retiring member to an erect, hard, imperious kinglike figure, standing as upright as a guardsman and as commanding as his fixed bayonet. When his penis is soft a man can be completely unaware that it exists; when it is erect, even when he is naked in a dark room, he cannot fail to be aware of its presence. Automatically his hand goes down, not merely to assure it of his awareness of it, but in the hopes of assuaging a little its swollen throbbing. Two or three minutes of the hand's attention and the man is submerged in the sweetest of all male human experiences.

When the woman is aroused, her state is not so blatantly brought to her attention, or, in fact, to the attention of anyone who observes her. Her vaginal lips swell but their covering of hair makes the swelling undetectable visually except at very close quarters, and though her clitoris becomes erect and emerges from its hood, it remains hidden from view by the folds of the outer lips. Though sensations accompany the swelling, according to the dozen or so women I have questioned, except on intermittent occasions, their diffuseness detracts from their intensity and attention to the affected swollen parts is not so directly directed as it is in the case of the man to his penis. While the man's touching of his penis is almost a reflex reaction, the touching of her vaginal lips and clitoris is a much more deliberate act on the part of the woman.

Nor do the differences end here. If the man is sexually aroused by the chemical reactions that take place within his body—as I shall be explaining in a moment—and not by his deliberate, direct stimulation of the penis or as a result of cerebral stimulation by sexual thoughts or sights—his feelings of tension and more often than not his erection will not subside until he has had an ejaculation and orgasm. The reason for this is that under the influence of chemical reactions the seminal vesicles—two small reservoirs which store the sperm made by the testicles and which produce their own fluid in which the sperm swim—become so full that they have to be emptied. Supposing an average, healthy man has no other sexual outlet, this filling up of the seminal vesicles takes place every three days. The pressure of sperm plus seminal fluid on the seminal vesicles sets up sexual tension and the penis automatically becomes erect, and if the man does not then deliberately masturbate, the next time he goes to sleep he will have a spontaneous erection, and during the course of an erotic dream he will have a spontaneous ejaculation and orgasm.

Though the woman is also sexually roused by chemical reactions that take place within her body, the mechanism is not the same. As she does not ejaculate, she has no equivalent of the seminal vesicles to become overloaded and set up tension which can only be relieved by orgasm. While it is true that some women do have erotic dreams during which they experience orgasm, the experience is very very much less widespread and very very much less frequent than is the man's experience. Because of this, the woman's spontaneous sexual arousal and experience of sexual tension will subside in time without her having obtained an orgasm. Unlike the man, therefore, the woman is far less tempted to masturbate. When the woman does masturbate, she does so, more often than not, not in response to the buildup of sexual tension, but from encouragement from sexual thoughts, or a deliberate act carried out to experience the delights of orgasm sensations.*

Probably nowhere in the sexual experience of a man and woman are their differences in sexual response so marked as in their masturbating activities. Large numbers of boys masturbate before they are ten years old. Admittedly, quite a number are initiated by older brothers or friends, but the majority have discovered it for themselves. Having had their attention directed to their penis by erection, they have touched it and played with it until they have come, because though boys cannot ejaculate, they can experience orgasm before they reach puberty. Boys are capable of erection within a short time of birth, and though no one can be certain of the earliest age at

*So that I shall not be misunderstood, there are women who do masturbate in response to chemically induced sexual tension, but they are only a fraction of the number of men who do so.

which they can experience orgasm, many authorities believe, from their observation of baby boys, that they are capable of orgasm as soon as they are capable of erection. I have myself observed a number of baby boys of between eighteen months and three years playing with their penises, and deriving obvious pleasure from it. (Boys, of course, cannot have chemically induced erections or build-up of sexual tension until they are past puberty. When baby boys have erections they are either due to irritation of the penis head, which causes the baby to handle his penis and bring about erection, or he has discovered the pleasure obtained from playing with his penis quite by chance, and subsequently repeats the experience deliberately.) Baby girls do not develop the same pattern of fondling their genitals and this pattern is carried over into adolescence.

It is an established fact that 99 percent of *all* boys masturbate with a fair measure of regularity before they have reached late adolescence, say seventeen. During these years, masturbation is their chief sexual outlet. As they have more opportunity for sexual intercourse, they masturbate with less frequency, but most men masturbate all their lives.

In contrast, it is an equally established fact that though the various authorities differ as to percentages, far fewer girls masturbate in adolescence. Kinsey puts the figure at 20 percent (as compared with the boys' 99 percent) by late adolescence, and with a fairly irregular frequency. The percentage increases during the middle twenties, and somewhat strangely, some may think, the highest percentage is reached between the ages of forty and fifty.

The Victorians took a frightening view of masturbation, especially male masturbation. Though I am not quite a Victorian, I was, however, brought up in this respect according to Victorian thinking on the subject. When I was informed of the facts of life at puberty I was told that masturbation was not only a sin, because it wasted God's most precious gift—human seed—but that if I did it I would have bad health, my brain would not function properly so that I should fail at my lessons, and I would be poor at games, because the waste of semen sapped one's energy. If I persisted in it, I would eventually go mad, I was assured. I was further frightened off by a story that the masturbator carried signs of his filthy, degrading, disgusting, weakening, and sinful habit of self-abuse on his face, signs known only to grownups, who, when they saw him would have nothing to do with him. No decent person would.

Though it was based on ignorance—the Victorians believed that if semen was not lost through masturbation, it would go into the bloodstream and enrich the health of the whole body, whereas we now know that this cannot possibly happen—it was an attitude which caused much unhappiness and suffering, not only in adolescence, but throughout adult life. For it set up feelings of guilt, sin, and shame which were carried over into adult sexual behavior—normal, adult, heterosexual behavior—which prevented the sex lives of far too many from being either normal or natural.

Now, because girls do not produce an ejaculate when they have an orgasm, such arguments could not be used to prevent them from "indulging in *the* secret vice." Nevertheless, they were warned off. Any mother who came upon her daughter fingering her "private parts," or had reason to believe that she might be doing so, threatened her with the most dire punishment if she ever caught her doing so, or believed that she might be doing so. A part of these warnings nearly always included a sermon on the filthiness of sex, even between husband and wife; that sex was something horrible which men were disgusting enough to be interested in, and something which no "nice" woman should ever allow herself to enjoy. It was a wifely duty to submit to men's sexual approaches, but only because men had ordained that it should be so, and because it was—regrettably—the only way in which women could fulfill their mother instincts.

The result of this attitude toward women's masturbating was, in the sum, no less psychologically devastating than the threats that were poised over men's heads in Damocleansword fashion. It was filthy, degrading, and sinful, and it would transform any girl who succumbed to it into a dehumanized woman.

Nowadays, of course, we have a far more complete understanding of the body's sexual functioning. We know that in the case of boys, the semen is what is known as an "external" secretion; that is, a secretion which does not and cannot enter the bloodstream whatever else happens to it; and that, on this account, it cannot affect the health. This point has had a tremendous influence on the whole concept of male masturbation, and since it is recognized, in this case at all events, that what is sauce for the gander is sauce also for the goose, on the concept of female masturbation also.

Far from being a menace to health, masturbation is actually physically beneficial. The sexual apparatus, like all other parts of the body, requires exercise to keep it in trim and toned up. But this is only of secondary importance to the tremendous psychological and emotional benefits that derive from it.

Because of their sexual chemistry men who are deprived of the opportunity for regular sexual intercourse must have some sexual outlet, otherwise the unreleased tensions will eventually lead to frustrations building up which will have an effect on the whole sexual function. I don't want to go into detail about this here as it affects the male, but denial of a sexual outlet of any kind can set up all kinds of psychological barriers which prevent him from having satisfactory and satisfying sexual relations with a woman. Though the unused semen will be automatically expelled from the body when the seminal vesicles become overfull, the orgasms achieved during these so-called "wet dreams" are not so psychically releasing as orgasms obtained consciously during masturbation.

This applies far more to the woman's experience of sex. Though the woman's sex drive and sexual desire are also derived from the promptings of certain of the sex hormones, which do not act in quite the same way as the man's, nor apparently with the same frequency—a number of authorities have shown that whereas the average male sexual desire is active three or four times a *week*, the average female sexual desire is active only two or three times a *month*—the woman feels the need of a sexual outlet that will satisfy her not only physically but psychologically as well. If she does not provide this outlet, in the absence of opportunity for intercourse, by masturbation, she, too, sets up psychological barriers which will inevitably affect her mature sexual functioning.

If physical and psychological benefits are derived from masturbation—and of this all authorities are agreed there is no doubt—what of that other old bogey which, in the past, has always reared its head wherever masturbation has been considered? I mean sin and immorality.

While I have been able to understand the concept of masturbation as being sinful with regard to males, I have never understood how it could possibly be applied to female masturbatory activities. It could be argued—but only so long as contraception was not recognized by the

Church of England and the nonconformist Churches—that the ejaculation of semen for any means but producing a baby was sinful in that it did divert "God's most precious gift" from its major use. As soon as contraception was recognized, however, this concept of masturbatory sin had to be eliminated, because the man who ejaculated into a condom, or into a vagina protected by other forms of contraceptive devices, was equally diverting his semen from its major use—the fertilization of the woman's egg. It was the realization of this that eventually resolved for me my very heavy burden of this particular sin. I had been given the dire warnings, but try as I might I could not resist all my urges to masturbate, and when I did "fall from grace" I suffered a mental agony which no adult, let alone young adolescent boy, should be required to suffer. After two or three years of such suffering, a kind, older friend was able to convince me that masturbation is not sinful.

This argument about wasting "God's most precious gift" could not be applied to female masturbation because when the woman masturbates she experiences sensations only; she does *not* ejaculate in any shape or form. Her equivalent to the male's loss of semen—the shedding of the unfertilized egg—was a biological function (menstruation) over which she had no control whatsoever. Yet, she was told that masturbation was sinful and was threatened with the most terrible consequences if she indulged.

Little girls, if left on their own, and who do not come under the influence of older girls, do not have the same curiosity about their genitals as little boys have about their penises. Those adolescent girls who do discover masturbation for themselves nearly always do so by accident. Irritation of the vaginal lips leads to rubbing for relief, and the rubbing, they find, not only relieves the irritation, but produces extremely pleasant sensations, which, if the rubbing is continued long enough, produce in their turn an explosion of sensations that are indescribably voluptuous. Many a girl has been introduced to orgasm by horse-riding and bicycle-riding, having realized that the saddle friction has caused it and that the friction can be produced in other ways. It is a fact, however, that quite a number of girls who masturbate are shown how to do so by older girls.

Except in cases where the mother has come upon the girl "playing with herself" or suspects that she may be doing so, girls are not warned, as a rule, about the sinfulness of masturbation until they are given their first general instruction about the facts of life, which generally happens between fourteen and fifteen, even when menstruation has taken place as early as twelve or thirteen. In the past, before sex instructions was given in schools, the majority of girls were given no instructions at all. Yet most girls who masturbated felt that what they were doing they must do in secret and keep secret. This attitude quickly developed tremendous feelings of guilt and shame, for which no rational explanation could be given. Nevertheless, more often than not these feelings build up into problems which afflict many women all their lives. The tragedy of it is that it all so unnecessary. Let me state quite categorically that the rules for masturbation for men apply equally for women! *Masturbation is neither sinful nor immoral and will do no physical harm! It is, on the contrary, psychologically beneficial!* These rules apply to all times of life. The mature woman who has no other sexual outlet has, in fact, a need to masturbate from time to time, for as she grows more physically mature, so her sex drive makes greater demands on her. Whereas in adolescence and young adulthood her sexual desire may subside if she does not satisfy it physically, as the years go by her frustrations will mount each time she tries to ignore it. Physical relief, in some form or other, becomes essential, and if opportunities for intercourse are not available, then masturbation is the best substitute. Providing no feelings of guilt or shame are connected with it—*and I stress, there is no reason whatsoever why there should be*—the physical relief will have only a beneficial psychological effect.

Women who have masturbated in adolescence often have quite the wrong ideas about the consequences. A young woman wrote to me recently:

Dear Mr. Chartham: Please will you help me with some advice. I am 23 years old and have just become engaged. We are to be married in six months, but I am very worried about several things. You see, I have been masturbating two or three times a week ever since I was thirteen, when a cousin showed me how to do it. My husband-to-be is a good, honest, and decent man, and I know he would be horrified if he knew that I had been engaging in this practice, which I know is horrible though I haven't been able to give it up however much I've tried.

MASTURBATION

Please can you tell me, will my husband be able to tell that I have been doing it for so long? I mean, will I have deformed myself in any way so that he will know by looking at me? Then, will the fact that I have been masturbated so long and so frequently have any effect on my enjoyment of sex with my husband after we are married? Lastly, will I have harmed myself in any way that could stop me having children, or will the children be deformed in any way?

Maybe this is an example of total ignorance about the effects that masturbation has, but it does represent vividly the misunderstanding that very many women have about physical sexual functioning. No matter how long or how frequently a woman has masturbated, except by one particular method, to which I will refer presently, no malformation of the clitoris, vaginal lips, or vaginal entrance will result. The one method which might, in fact, almost invariably does, cause a physical change is a very rarely used method indeed. There are a few women, very few, who masturbate not by stimulating the clitoris directly but by pulling on the vaginal lips. This pulling and releasing of the vaginal lips has the same effect on these organs as the in-and-out-thrusting of the penis in the vagina during normal intercourse. As the penis is pushed deep into the vagina it pulls on the vaginal lips, which in turn pulls the clitoral hood down over the clitoris; as the penis is drawn back, it releases the pressure on the vaginal lips and the clitorial hood slides back over the clitoris. This is what happens when the woman masturbates by pulling on the vaginal lips. Because the action of the clitoral hood sliding backwards and forwards over the clitoris is a very gentle one, it takes a long time for the woman to reach orgasm by this method. If she begins to masturbate in this way in early adolescence and does so once or twice a week, in a year or two the vaginal lips become permanently stretched and protuberant. (Some African tribes regard protuberant vaginal lips physically attractive and sexually stimulating, and mothers begin to stretch their daughters' for a short time daily from very early childhood.) As I have said, not many women do masturbate in this way, and I doubt very much if the average man would take any notice of protuberant vaginal lips, or if he did would put it down to masturbation. As with the penis, so with the woman's genitalia; though the general conformation is the same, there are so many detailed differences that there are very few that are exactly identical. None of the other methods by which a woman can masturbate do cause physical changes to take place, so it is impossible for a man to tell whether his partner has masturbated or not.

The other two questions have equally negative answers. In the vast majority of cases, masturbatory activity at any age does not interfere with subsequent sexual function or enjoyment of sex. Certainly, masturbation by whatever method cannot prevent or give rise to difficulties of conception, nor can it harm future children in any way.

One other difference between the male and female experience of masturbation lies in the variety of methods open to the female and the lack of variety open to the male. The man invariably concentrates on providing his penis with friction of some kind or another. In fact, 98 percent of men are unaware that they can bring themselves to orgasm by placing a firm object, like a small box or a book, high up between their thighs behind the scrotum and merely squeezing their thighs about the object, not touching the penis at all. However, this method and two others—the stimulation of a sensitive anal sphincter by a vibrator or the manipulation of highly sensitive nipples, both of which will only work for individuals who are abnormally sensitive in these areas—are the only ways in which men can masturbate without applying direct friction to the penis.

Women, on the other hand, can bring themselves to orgasm by stimulating other areas besides the clitoris. Large numbers, especially in adolescence and early maturity, can bring themselves to orgasm by stimulating their nipples only, by reason of the fact that the nervous system of the breasts is directly connected with the female general nervous system. Others habitually masturbate by manipulating the vaginal lips, while for others the vaginal rim is so sensitive that by a rapid stroking of it with a finger or some object they gain a fairly easy orgasm. The anal sphincter of many women is also sensitive to the use of a vibrator, while the squeezing together of the thighs is one of the most common methods.

Now it is very, very rare indeed for a boy to develop difficulties in achieving orgasm in normal intercourse as an adult because of masturbation techniques he used in adolescence or is using in adulthood. Men do suffer from two types of sexual failure during intercourse, the most common of which is premature ejaculation, and much more rare, retarded ejaculation. Premature and too rapid ejaculation are what happens when the man is unable to control the speed of his progress towards orgasm, and he either ejaculates before he is able to get his penis into the vagina (premature ejaculation) or within a few seconds of putting the penis in the vagina (too rapid ejaculation). In both cases he is unable to satisfy his partner by bringing her to orgasm by penis-vagina contact, and when he does ejaculate too soon the accompanying orgasm is also of low and unsatisfying intensity. Retarded ejaculation is when, however long the man moves his penis in the vagina, he is unable to bring himself to orgasm. Men suffering from this condition can maintain their erections for up to an hour or longer, and yet however much they stimulate the penis cannot obtain an orgasm, which leaves them intolerably physically tensed and psychologically frustrated. Neither of these conditions, however, can be attributed to masturbatory activities, either to the technique of masturbation used or to frequency of masturbation.

Women, on the other hand, can have their experience of orgasm affected by their methods of masturbation. For example, those who use stimulation of the whole genital area with emphasis on the vaginal opening very rarely have difficulty in experiencing orgasm during penis-vagina contact in intercourse; in fact, large numbers of them report that they come at the very first attempt at intercourse. Those, on the other hand, who have masturbated for some years by direct stimulation of the clitoris only, have greater difficulty in making the transition from masturbation-orgasm to intercourse-orgasm. They do, of course, eventually achieve it, but it usually takes six months of regular intercourse and the cooperation of a sympathetic and patient partner in breaking down the feelings of guilt—which, if they have not been present during the adolescent masturbation, develop after the first few failures to reach orgasm during intercourse—and in replacing direct clitoral stimulation by other methods of stimulation, preferably by concentrating on the vaginal opening.

Other masturbatory habits also have an effect on the woman's achievement of orgasm during intercourse. I shall be referring to these in detail in the next chapter.

The young lady who wrote me the letter I have just quoted also revealed a very common misapprehension from which many women suffer—quite unnecessarily. In her fear that her fiancé might be able to tell that she had masturbated for some time, she showed that she believed that he would think the worse of her if he knew she had. In her particular case, knowing her fiancé as she did, she might have been right in her assumption, but for one puritanical and sexually ignorant man who might take exception, there are hundreds of thousands of men who would regard their partners as abnormal if they had never masturbated.

Women should read, mark, learn, and inwardly digest that for 99 percent of all men, masturbation is a part of their sexual nature, and a prominent part at that. It is true that some men—even young men in this day and age—still have feelings of guilt and shame about their masturbatory activities, but even these feelings do not prevent them from masturbating, while those who do not have these feelings regard the activity as so essential a part of their sex lives that they take it for granted that their partners have had the same experience. Countless men have told me that they prefer their partners to have had masturbatory experience, for they do at least then know what they ought to expect. Some men have even told me that if they had known that their partners had not masturbated, they would not have formed a relationship. In putting forward these views I am not intending to encourage women to masturbate who have not discovered it for themselves. What I am trying to stress is that there is no need for any woman who has masturbated to conceal the fact from her husband or partner.

One very good reason why a woman should tell her partner is that if she masturbated she is almost certain to have experimented to discover which techniques of stimulation arouse her most. No matter how skilled a lover her partner may be, he cannot possibly know this by instinct. He may discover them by experiment, but it is equally on the cards that he may not. Not only will it save time if she tells him straightaway when to stimulate her and how, it will also save her a good deal of frustration. Many women quite needlessly suffer agonies of unrelieved tension simply because they will not tell their lovers what to do. If he is a wise lover he will ask, but if he doesn't ask, don't hesitate to tell him and show him. If it will embarrass you less, ask him what he most likes to have done to him. He will be grateful to you for asking, because though he may come round to it in time, he may hold back out of deference to the fact that you are a woman.

Many women are worried about their own and particularly about their husband's masturbation after marriage. Masturbation is quite normal for both partners in a number of situations. For example, during temporary absences it would be abnormal if both did not masturbate, and it would be equally strange, if the partner could not supply full relief by lovemaking, not to make up the deficit by masturbation. Where there has been a row during which such things have been said that a reconciliation, sealed by lovemaking, does not seem immediately possible to either partner, it is natural to use masturbation to avoid sexual tension.

What is not appreciated by many women, however, is that very large numbers of happily married men, who are entirely satisfied sexually by their lovemaking, also masturbate from time to time. I have a bulging file of letters from wives who have discovered that the husband whom they believed they were completely satisfying masturbates, too. They complain that the discovery has been a terrific shock. As one woman, speaking for many, puts it, "It has made me feel sexually inadequate. Where have I gone wrong? What can I do?"

You have not gone wrong anywhere, and what you can do is to understand that your husband is in no way criticizing you. As I have explained earlier, men are sexually roused extremely easily and rapidly, and can be just as rapidly relieved by masturbating. Two or three minutes' manipulation of the erect penis is all that is necessary. Take, for instance, a Sunday morning. You may have made love on waking, then after a pleasant lie-in, you get up and get dressed and go downstairs to get breakfast, leaving your husband to follow when you are ready. Even though he has been completely satisfied by your lovemaking, this does not preclude his getting another erection and feeling sexually tense. It may even have been triggered off by his savoring the experience of only a half hour or so ago. As he is a thoughtful husband, he won't call down to you to stop your chores, come upstairs and get undressed. Yet he has to have relief from his present tensions, he knows he can obtain it in a couple of minutes or so, so he provides himself with it. Or, he may be in the bath. The sensation of warm water lapping over the body has a sexually arousing effect on many men, resulting in erection and tension. Unless he is bathing immediately before going to bed, it would not be very thoughtful of him to demand you leave whatever you are doing and get into the bath with him, would it?

If you enjoy a happy and satisfying sex life, you cannot possibly be sexually inadequate simply because your husband—especially if he is uncircumcised—masturbates from time to time, even as frequently as once or twice a week. Nor, knowing how he can react in this way, will he accuse himself of being inadequate sexually for you, if he knows you masturbate now and again.

I repeat: masturbation is second (sexual) nature to most men. There is no reason why it should not be so for you. Certainly you are creating difficulties where none need exist if, when prompted to masturbate, you do not take it in your stride.

Chapter TWO

Frigidity and Pseudo-frigidity

No other aspect of human sexual response is so misunderstood as the condition which afflicts women known as frigidity.

Dear Mr. Chartham: Please can you help me? I am frigid and it is worrying both me and my husband very much. For the last two and a half years I have never reached climax during lovemaking. We have been married nine years and have two lovely children aged seven and five, and for the first six and a half years of our marriage our sex life was perfect. My husband always was a wonderful lover, but as the years went by he became more and more wonderful, and there was never a time when we made love that I didn't come, sometimes two or three times. Then I don't know what happened. Gradually I seemed to lose all my sensitivity, and whatever he did (and does), though I get very aroused, he just cannot get me over the top. I get to a certain point when I think it's going to be all right, but then I get stuck there and can go no further. It is beginning to affect our whole relationship. It makes me terribly tensed up and frustrated, and if I couldn't masturbate, which I can do fairly easily, I don't know what I would do. But, all the same, this is a very poor substitute for the real thing. And my poor husband! He has got it into his head that he's lost his touch, and that he is inadequate for me sexually. I try to tell him that this just isn't true, but I'm afraid it doesn't help him. I get touchy and snap at him sometimes for absolutely no reason at all, and he snaps back. We never used to do this and it is making us both very miserable, and as I say, is spoiling our whole relationship. I am only thirty; surely I can't have lost my ability to have satisfying sex? We've both been to see our doctor but he doesn't seem to understand; he says this sort of thing often happens for a short time, and that everything will come out all right. But to me two and a half years isn't a short time, it seems more like a lifetime. Please, Mr. Chartham, what can we do? You are our only hope.

This unhappy young woman has a problem, *but she is not frigid!*

Dear Mr. Chartham: I am very unhappy because I've lost all interest in sex, and it is making my husband very unhappy, too. I am twenty-four and my husband is twenty-six. We have been married two years and haven't any children, yet, though we are planning to have some.

I used to enjoy making love quite as much as Roger did to begin with. In fact, sometimes he used to say I was going sex-mad because some periods of the month I would want to make love two or three times a day. Now I never want to make love. Of course I let Roger make love to me, and he nearly always makes me come. But when I come, it isn't half so good as it used to be, and if he didn't make love to me when he felt like it, I'd never make love at all. Even when he does make love to me, I feel at the beginning that I wish he would be quick and get it over with. When we first got married, we generally used to make love for an hour or more, and I enjoyed and got a terrific thrill out of every minute of it. And I used to enjoy making love to him. He taught me how to caress his penis with my mouth, and from the very first time I tried it, I found it very exciting and always wanted to do it to him. But now I can't even be bothered to rouse myself to bend over him to do it. Is there any hope of my getting my old enjoyment of lovemaking back? I do hope so, because Roger has noticed how changed I am and thinks it is something to do with him. I don't know how long he will put up with me if I can't pull myself together. Can you help me?

FRIGIDITY AND PSEUDO-FRIGIDITY   31

This young woman, too, has a problem, *but she is not frigid, either!*

True frigidity is when a woman *has never in her life* felt any sexual drive, and has never in her life been stimulated to orgasm. Such cases, like male organically caused impotence, are very very rare indeed.

The two cases referred to in the letters I have quoted are what I call pseudo-frigidity. The first woman cannot possibly be frigid, because although she does not reach orgasm as a result of any stimulation her husband applies to her, she can bring herself to orgasm if she masturbates. The truly frigid woman could not masturbate to climax, but as this woman can reach orgasm, obviously there cannot be any organic reason for her not being able to reach climax during lovemaking. She represents the classic case of pseudo-frigidity, the inability to reach orgasm during intercourse resulting from psychological causes, though what the specific cause is in this particular case it is not possible to say, and would only become apparent during face-to-face counseling. Even then the counselor might not be able to discover it because it was too deeply hidden in the subconscious, in which event, psychotherapy would hold the only possibility of cure.

The first reaction of most women who come to me for help because they are unable to come during lovemaking is to deny, when I suggest it, that they have any reason at all, and certainly not a psychological reason, for withholding their orgasm, because that is what is basically happening. Some become quite worked up about it and protest that they are surprised that I can suggest any such thing.

The layman, and, indeed, a good many doctors who do not specialize in sexual problems, has no idea the power that the mind exerts over our *physical* sexual functioning. Men are as much at the mercy of their minds as women are. For example, fewer than 5 percent of all cases of total impotence, i.e., when the man cannot get an erection at all, have organic causes; the remainder of the cases have psychological causes. *All* cases of partial impotence—when the man can get an erection, but the erection subsides during loveplay, or just as he is about to put the penis in the vagina, or within seconds of getting it in the vagina, or, in a few cases where the penis will only become semi-stiff, not stiff enough to get into the vagina—*all* these cases have psychological causes. So have 98 percent of all cases of premature ejaculation—when the man comes before he can get the penis into the vagina—

ADVICE TO WOMEN

and 99 percent of all cases of retarded ejaculation (when the man can obtain an erection and hold it for an hour or more, but no matter how long he stimulates his penis, he cannot achieve orgasm).

Let me give an example of the ease with which the mind affects the physical functioning of a man. Ethel and George were not lucky enough to get a house before they married, and as Ethel's parents had a spare room, it was decided that the couple should live there for a few months while they continued their search.

One Sunday, after they had been married for two or three weeks, while having a lie-in they began to make love. Eventually they coupled, and George had not been in operation more than two or three minutes, when both of them were startled to hear a boyish voice near them, demanding, "Hi, George, what are you doing to Ethel?" George naturally reared off Ethel like a horse stung by a hornet, and they looked round to see Ethel's eight-year-old brother, Freddie, standing by the bed. They had been so engrossed in their lovemaking that they had not heard the boy come into the room.

They shooed him away and tried to restart their lovemaking, having first made sure that the door of their room was locked. Fortunately they were young and they soon began to respond to one another's caresses. Unfortunately, within seconds of coupling, however, George lost what had been a very presentable erection before he could come himself or bring Ethel to climax. No matter how hard they tried George could not sustain his rigidity once he had coupled. And so it happened every time they made love, though they took good care always to lock their bedroom door, and knew they could not possibly be interrupted. (Happily they were both fairly uncomplicated, and were able to relieve each other's tensions by heavy petting.) Not until they moved into their own flat five months later was George able to function normally again.

Then there was Maud. Maud and her boyfriend were making love in lush grass in a secluded corner of a field one pleasant summer evening. They had coupled and were beginning to speed pleasurably toward the point-of-no-return when they heard a man's voice bellowing above them, "You filthy souls! Don't you know it is against God's laws to fornicate? You whore of Babylon ...!" The young man had begun to come just as the angry old man spoke and nothing could stop him. Maud was not so lucky and every time thereafter, whenever they made love, even in the security of a hotel bedroom, she failed to come. She had her first orgasm during coupling on her wedding night. The old man's moral strictures had bitten much more deeply into her subconscious than she would have admitted. As soon as the wedding ring was on her finger, and she could no longer be guilty of fornication, all was well.

There was Tom, too. Tom, aged ten, went swimming one day in a lake. They had no bathing suits, but that did not deter them, nor did the coldness of the water. After a time, when they had swum enough, they began to fool about and soon the older boys initiated a mutual masturbation session. Tom had heard about this pastime, but had no idea of the mechanics of it. One of the other boys soon put him wise, giving him a practical demonstration, with the result that Tom had his very first orgasm standing at the edge of the lake with his feet in cold water.

He came to see me sixteen years later. He had been two years married but he still could not come unless he had his feet in cold water. He never had been able to.

"How on earth do you manage, then?" I asked him.

"Well," he said, "I sit on the edge of the bath with my feet in cold water, and she sits astride me. It's the only way we can make love satisfactorily and she's getting fed up. In fact, unless something happens pretty soon, I think she will leave me."

It was a case, of course, for real expert psychotherapy. It takes a little time fixing up such treatment, and, in a sudden flash of inspiration (!) I suggested that while he was waiting, he should try filling a plastic bag with ice cubes, and when coupling in bed, he should put his feet on the bag. I must admit that I made the suggestion more or less tongue-in-cheek, and I never expected any results at all. My letter telling him of the arrangements I had made for him to have a course of psychotherapy crossed with one from him which read:

Dear Robert: I hope you don't mind me calling you that. I shan't need to visit your psychiatrist. We did as you suggested with the ice cubes in a plastic bag, and it worked first time, though it did make the bed a bit of a mess, because the bag leaked. After two or three times with the bag, we decided to do without it to see what happened. AND IT WORKED! We can now couple in all the positions you describe in *Husband & Lover*, and more besides, and I come every time. I can come, too, when Eve fellates me. I could only ever do that before, though it aroused me terrifically, unless I was standing in the bath. We just don't know how to thank you. We are both quite certain we would have split up if I hadn't been "cured." Our very sincere thanks.

Yours ever, Tom.

I have quoted these three cases at this length in order to demonstrate how powerful the mind is over physical sexual functioning in both men and women, and also to show that strange and often momentary occurrences can have a really devastating effect on us. Many of the psychological causes of pseudo-frigidity are just as odd, and some so at odds with the conscious attitudes of the woman toward her partner that maybe there will be some of you reading this who will not be able to believe some of the causes I shall be setting out. Before I go on to these psychological causes, however, there are two particular types of pseudo-frigidity which have neither an organic cause in the sense that there is something wrong with the formation of the woman's sexual apparatus or a fault in her sexual nervous system, nor a psychological cause.

The first type was being experienced by the woman who wrote the second letter I quoted at the beginning of the chapter. When I put further questions to her, I discovered that she was on the Pill, and had been so for the past three and a half years.

Until comparatively recently I have been puzzled by a number of cases of young wives who come to me complaining that when they had first got married they and their husbands had had very satisfying and very happy sex lives. Then gradually—it was usually at the end of twelve to fifteen months of being married—they had begun to lose all interest in sex, and now found themselves in the very same circumstances as the writer of the letter, without sexual desire, not caring whether their husbands made love to them or not, yet nearly always coming at the culmination of lovemaking.

It did not occur to me at first that there might be any connection between the Pill and this loss of interest in sex, but the incidence of Pill-taking plus the loss of sexual desire and interest in lovemaking was too high to be coincidence. In the last seven weeks, for example, I have had no fewer than twelve cases of young wives between the ages of twenty and twenty-four, married two or three years, who went on the Pill at marriage and who after a year to fifteen months of sexual bliss now do not care if their husbands make love to them or not.

Not all women on the Pill are afflicted in this way; on the other hand it is not one brand of Pill that is responsible, but several brands.

I now do not hesitate, when confronted with such a case, in urging the woman to go to her doctor, explain what has happened to her, insist that she comes off the Pill and ask to be fitted with an IUD instead, or some other contraceptive device. It takes a good six months for these side-effects of the Pill to wear off, but sexual desire, interest, and normal functioning is eventually restored. All that is needed is patience from both partners and sympathy and understanding from the husband—who, poor devil, has already had the shock of wondering whether he had become sexually inadequate for his partner.

The following is a typical letter I receive:

Dear Robert Chartham: I have been married eight years and have never had an orgasm during lovemaking, though I can come fairly easily if I masturbate. We went to our doctor a year or two ago, but he was more embarrassed than we were, and all he told us was that some women never do reach orgasm during intercourse and we would just have to make the best of it. . . .

It took me quite a long time to realize that some cases of pseudo-frigidity unconnected with the Pill do not have psychological causes. Now I have worked out a routine to which I work if the letters I receive do not *at once* reveal a possible psychological cause, and I feel certain that even the experts would be surprised by the number of women who are deprived of orgasm during lovemaking by the sheer ignorance of themselves or their partner, and by the faulty loveplay techniques of the partner.

When I receive a letter like the one I have just quoted, I write back and say, "Please tell me, (1) who decides when your partner puts his penis into you? You or him? (2) If you ask him to come into you, are you absolutely sure that you have let him stimulate you long enough? (3) If he decides without asking you if you are ready, do you wish he would stimulate you longer before he comes into you?"

It is quite fantastic the number of intelligent couples where the decision to couple is left to the husband, who makes no reference to the wife as to whether or not she is sufficiently roused. And almost invariably in these cases the wife wishes that she could be stimulated longer before penis-entry.

The whole object of loveplay is to close what I call the arousal-gap by bringing the woman to the *threshold of the point-of-no-return,* that point at which she feels that if the man continues to stimulate her for another few seconds she will come, before the penis is put into the vagina. The woman of experience should be able to judge this point to a nicety; and if any woman reading this cannot do so, she and her husband should experiment until she can. The number of women who are unable to judge this point is really quite surprising, and, in consequence, even when the decision for penis-entry is left to the woman, in many cases she has not let herself be sufficiently stimulated by loveplay.

If the woman has not been sufficiently stimulated during loveplay she will rarely come by penis-vagina contact, even if the man can swing his penis backwards and forwards in the vagina for fifteen, twenty, or perhaps thirty minutes without coming himself. Very many women require continued stimulation of the clitoral area by a finger or some other means during coupling, if she is to come while the penis is moving inside her. Yet so few couples make any attempt to supply this stimulation.

Once the decision to couple has been taken, even assuming that the woman has been sufficiently stimulated and brought to the threshold of the point-of-no-return, not a second should be wasted in getting the penis into the vagina. This is a much more difficult operation than women suppose, and to make it easier the woman should reach down between her legs, spread the vaginal lips, and guide the penis to the vaginal entrance.

It is essential that no time should be lost for this reason. Very many women indeed require continued clitoral stimulation right to orgasm. A five-second pause, and the arousal sensations fall right back; a couple of seconds more and she is right back where she started—unroused. If she is to come with the penis in the vagina, then the man must devise some way of stimulating the clitoris after coupling. (I shall be explaining how this can be done in the following chapter.) Fortunately the woman whose sensations have fallen back does not need such a long

FRIGIDITY AND PSEUDO-FRIGIDITY

stimulation to bring her on a second time. But if she is not so stimulated, then she will not come.

Many a woman has gone through her married life without having an orgasm during coupling for these reasons. The first thing the woman who has never experienced intercourse orgasm should do, therefore, is to examine the stimulation techniques she and her partner employ, and then make the necessary adjustments. She will soon cease to be pseudo-frigid!

I am sometimes asked by women who can come by masturbation but not during lovemaking whether earlier masturbatory activities can be the cause of pseudo-frigidity. In 99.9 percent of cases the answer is a definite No. There is the odd case, however, of the girl who began to masturbate at twelve or thirteen, and who has masturbated very frequently—and by *frequently* I mean daily or nearly daily—and regularly ever since. Such women generally develop special masturbation techniques, some of which do actually desensitize the clitoral nerve system or condition it to the extent that only the specific technique will bring on orgasm. Generally when this happens all arousal sensitivity is centered on the clitoris, and only by stimulation of the clitoris in the special way to which it has long been accustomed will the woman achieve orgasm. She will never come during penis-vagina contact; only by masturbation.

But even this type of pseudo-frigidity can be overcome. A new area of sensitivity has to be developed. It is usually the vagina entrance, but I have known cases when the perineum (which lies between the vagina entrance and the anus) and the anal sphincter have become so sensitive that they have quite deflated the clitoris' ego. I would, however, stress again that *this kind of case is very very rare*.

So now, what about psychologically caused pseudo-frigidity?

There are so many different causes, that I can only list the most common ones. First, there is the woman who fears unwanted pregnancy. Though she may be roused and be brought to the threshold of the point-of-no-return, as soon as the penis is put into her she goes tense, and no amount of stimulation while the penis is in the vagina will bring her to orgasm. Adopting the IUD or the Pill as the method of birth control, so that she can be as sure as little green apples that she will not become pregnant, overcomes the pseudo-frigidity in many cases; so will the sterilization of the husband by vasectomy, though I have had two complaints from sterilized husbands that their wives' pseudo-frigidity has not subsequently disappeared. I feel pretty certain that in these cases there has been additional psychological cause besides the fear of pregnancy. By far the largest group of women who suffer from this type of pseudo-frigidity are to be found among those whose husbands use *coitus interruptus,* the "withdrawal" method of birth control. I have known several cases where even the use of a condom has overcome the fear and the woman has experienced orgasm regularly thereafter.

Then there is the woman who has thoroughly enjoyed sex and may even have multiple orgasms and who then has a difficult time during the birth of her first child. She would like to opt out of sex altogether if she could, but she realizes she must keep her husband happy sexually, so lets him make love to her. But because she takes part in lovemaking, it isn't to say that she enjoys it. In fact, to prove to herself that she does not, she denies herself the experience of orgasm.

Another quite common psychological cause for pseudo-frigidity is the wife's resentment of her husband. This resentment generally lies very deep in the subconscious, and the woman when taxed with it will honestly, sincerely, and quite fiercely deny it. But take the case of Maureen.

Before she married Peter, Maureen had a very responsible job as personal assistant to a very prominent industrialist. Peter was also in business, was more than likely to make his mark, and was ambitious. He had been brought up to believe that wives should not have an outside job, that a man should be able to support a wife or not marry. Because she loved him, Maureen happily gave up her job.

For the first eighteen months, their sex lives were happy and satisfying. Then she developed pseudo-frigidity. Their doctor told them this happened sometimes, and that she would be all right again if she had a baby. She said she did not want a baby yet, but Peter insisted. After it was born, the pseudo-frigidity did not disappear.

When they seemed to be on the point of breaking up, they came to me. I sensed at once Maureen's resentment of Peter, and when I put it to her she hotly denied it. But when I insisted that I was right and explained why, she agreed.

What had happened was that after some months of marriage, Maureen had begun to be bored at home and wished she was back at her job. No sooner did she wish so, than she began to tell herself that if Peter hadn't been so old fashioned and forbidden her to work, she might now be a junior executive herself, with a bright future before her. This sparked off her resentment which grew stronger the more successful in business Peter became. It increased even more after the baby was born, because she felt trapped.

In her resentment, she decided to punish Peter by preventing him from satisfying her sexually. She determined to make him feel sexually inadequate.

Taking Peter on one side I explained all this to him, and he was horrified.

"But if I'd known she was as keen on her job as all that, I wouldn't have asked her to give it up," he exclaimed. "What's to be done?"

"I suggest you tell her now that if she wants to go back to work, as soon as young Christopher is weaned you'll engage a nanny," I said.

He did so, and the effect was dramatic. Within a day or two Maureen's pseudo-frigidity had disappeared. But she never did return to work. Just the knowledge that she could do so if she wished was enough to remove her resentment, and her desire to punish Peter.

Other causes of pseudo-frigidity take us into more abstruse psychological realms. There is the girl who falls in love with her father, and so idealizes him that no other man can match up to him. She shows her disdain of the inferior man by refusing fully to cooperate with him sexually. Or there is the girl whose mother, because of an unhappy experience of sex, has brought her up to regard sex as disgusting. She must marry, either because it is a status symbol, or for security, but she will never cooperate sexually with her husband. Or there is the unhappy girl, who as a child had an unpleasant sexual experience, and imagines all sex to be like that.

So I could go on, but I think I have shown how diverse the psychological causes of pseudo-frigidity are. The chief thing to remember is that *all pseudo-frigidity can be "cured"* if only the victim is herself patient and her partner is sympathetic and fully cooperative.

Chapter THREE

"My Husband Doesn't Know How to Rouse Me!"

When I read this sentence in a letter a young wife wrote to me not long ago, my first reaction was, "Then teach him how to, madam!" But the more I thought about it, the more I realized that though this was how the problem ought to be solved, in many cases it was easier to propose than to act upon.

Dear Dr. Chartham [she wrote]: I am twenty-two and my husband is twenty-four. Before we got married I was a nurse, and my husband, who is a truck driver, was one of my patients. That is how we got to know one another. He's a handsome man, slim, not an ounce of fat on him, and very strong. He is also what is known, I believe, as well-equipped sexually, and he can keep his erection indefinitely so it seems. He can come into me and keep up his movements for twenty minutes to half an hour before he comes. But that is not long enough for me, because, you see, he never rouses me before he gets in me. He doesn't know how to rouse me!

You'll probably say, how do you know he doesn't know how to rouse you? As I want your help, and want it very badly, I have to be frank, but I hope that what I'm going to tell you now, Dave need never know: While I was training I had an affair with a young doctor. It was what you might call an affair of sexual convenience. He was engaged—he told me so quite honestly, the first time he made a pass at me—and I knew we shouldn't marry; but I was quite happy to let him make love to me twice or three times a week, because it was much nicer than masturbating, which I had been doing since I was about

40

thirteen. Though he was younger than Dave is now, he knew what to do. We used to spend two or three hours in bed, and he would never come into me the first time without playing with me for at least an hour, even if I asked him to. (I think he must have read your book.) He would bring me up to what you call the point-of-no-return and then stop for a while. After our first two or three times together, he made me tell him when to stop, and if I didn't and I went right over, as happened once or twice, he used to get really annoyed. He seemed to know everything in the book (some of the things he did shocked me at first, until I realized how lovely they made me feel) and once he had come in me he could hold back until I came, always twice. So you see, I do know what making love should be like.

Well, all Dave does to me is to play with and suck my nipples until they are hard. While he is doing that he puts his hand on my vulva and as soon as I am wet, he comes in me. As I say, he can keep going for twenty minutes to half an hour before coming. Every now and again he asks me if I am coming, and in sheer desperation I say yes. But I never do come. I wait until he has gone to sleep and masturbate.

He doesn't know anything about loveplay, I'm positive. I know you are going to say I must tell him about it. But how can I! It would hurt him to think I was criticizing him, and in any case he might want to know how I knew, and I couldn't tell him that, because that would hurt him, too, and if I didn't tell him, he would probably suspect, and that would be just as bad. So what *can* I do?

What, indeed?

It may strike the more sophisticated as odd that nowadays, despite all the books on lovemaking that are available at prices to suit everyone's pocket, there should still be young men like Dave who have no idea about loveplay and loveplay techniques. I used to be surprised, too, at first, but there is so much evidence to confirm Dave's wife's protest, that I am surprised no longer. Mind you, there are equally many, if not more, girls who are just as ignorant, and far too many who are married to ignorant husbands and who go through life wondering what all this cracked-up sex is all about. For many ignorant women, however, no problem arises, because they have had the good fortune to marry sexually sophisticated husbands who, by tradition, are expected to know all about lovemaking and are able to instruct their partners as a matter of course.

(I suppose most people know by this time that I am dead against this state of affairs. It is my firm view that all women ought to equip themselves at any rate with the *theory* of lovemaking before they marry. If they do, so much time can be saved, for the knowledgeable couple will adjust to one another much more quickly than they otherwise would. Women, too, have a role to play in physical sex, which is of equal importance with the man's. The ignorant women not only deprives herself of a richer sexual experience, but her partner as well.)

The experienced woman married to an ignorant man does pose a problem. My correspondent, Avis, was quite right when she said Dave would be hurt if he thought she was criticizing him. Strangely enough, ignorant men are very jealous of their traditional role as the sexual leader, and I am pretty certain Dave would be one of them. The more experienced a lover a man is, the more he welcomes suggestions from his partner, but a man who knows little can very quickly have what confidence he has got in his sexual ability undermined, and he will join the ranks of those sex problem-children, who believe themselves to be sexually inadequate for their partners.

Once a man gets the idea into his head that he is sexually inadequate, more often than not he presents himself, and his partner, with a lifetime of misery. It is possible to exorcise this false notion by psychotherapy, but it is a long job, requiring patience on the part of both, and sympathy, understanding, and patience on the part of the woman. I have been taken to task more than once for telling women to be careful not to wound their partner's sexual ego, but since my critics are obviously sexually unhappy women who have, more likely than not, brought about their own unhappiness in the way I am describing, I feel I must not be depressed for stating it again.

I have pointed out already how strange it is that compared with the simplicity of the male sexual apparatus and its functioning how vulnerable it is to the working of the mind and how many problems and difficulties it may develop. I am not exaggerating when I say that an involuntary exclamation by the partner at a crucial moment, a thoughtless comment on the size of the penis probably spoken half in jest, or a simple injunction to "hurry up and

DOESN'T KNOW HOW TO ROUSE ME!

get on with it," can and does strike a deep wound in a man's manhood. The letters on my files supporting this are among the more numerous of the cases of male sexual problems. If a woman wants to destroy her man sexually she need not lift a finger to do so; a word, a sound, a gesture is quite enough.

It all springs, of course, from the fact that man has always been regarded as the leader in sexual activity. He is the knowledgeable one, and on him depends the success of the lovemaking, according to the gospel of Dr. Marie Stopes and others. I feel quite sure that when a man judged his manhood by the strength of his erection rather than by his prowess as a lover, half his problems did not exist. I feel equally certain that the time will come again when more than half his problems have disappeared—the time when all women have accepted equal responsibilities and have become equal partners in lovemaking and men have acceded them this sexual equality. Though we are on the right road, we have still a long way to go, and while we are getting there we must look upon men as the sexually fragile creatures they really are.

David is one of these sexually fragile creatures, and probably without knowing why, Avis is aware of it. If she lets David know in terms that he cannot misunderstand that she is getting no joy, no satisfaction out of their lovemaking because he lacks a lover's skills, she will deprive herself of all hope of ever getting satisfaction and joy from their lovemaking. Once he is made to feel sexually inadequate, he will become sexually inadequate. So what *can* she do?

Whatever she does, she must do gradually. First, I suggest that she places her hand over the hand which he puts on her clitoral area when he begins to caress her, and moves it up and down. To indicate how pleasant she finds it, she can sigh or murmur some word of appreciation. If when he takes her hand away, he stops moving his hand, she can replace her own hand, whispering to him to go on a little longer because it is so good.

On the first occasion, after urging him on once, I think she must leave it to him to decide when to couple. She will probably be more frustrated at the end of it than she has been previously, but if he is at all quick on the uptake she shouldn't be frustrated after lovemaking for much longer. If he has taken the hint, the next time they make love he will move his hand on the clitoral area on his own initiative, but if he does not, then she must repeat the tactics of the first time, and this time she must insist that he does it until she is ready for him to go into her. She probably won't come this time, either, but she will have made some progress, for I am quite certain that on the third occasion, unless he is an imbecile (which I am sure he is not) or has a sizeable psychological block where loveplay is concerned (which is very rare, indeed), he will not have to be prompted to stimulate her clitoral area.

After he has been moving his hand a few minutes, this time she should part her vaginal lips, and taking one of his fingers, place it on or beside the clitoris, whichever provides her with the most stimulation—which she will know from her masturbation techniques—and ask him if he can feel her "little man," or some other appropriate name she may be able to think of for the clitoris. When he has felt it she should move his finger so that it stimulates her clitorally, and while doing so she should make even more appreciative sighs and sounds. If, when she takes her hand away he stops moving his finger, she should make it clear to him that she wants him to go on.

I am quite sure that when a man does not direct his attention to the clitoris during loveplay, it is because he has never heard of it. I am not inventing this, for twice within the past month I have had letters from couples asking me what the clitoris is and where it is located. Both couples had been married two or three years and their first encounter with the word was in the magazine *Forum*. (Obviously they had read no marriage manuals, and the wives had not used direct clitoral stimulation while masturbating, if, in fact, they had ever masturbated.) But he would be a very backward lover indeed who, once having located the clitoris and noted the effect stimulation of it could have on his partner, did not subsequently return to it.

Having cottoned on at last, he must now be encouraged to stimulate it until she has been brought to the threshold of the point-of-no-return. By this time, and having got him so far without any apparent injury to his sexual self-respect, I think she can tell him without any beating about the bush that she wants him to continue until she tells him to stop. I also think she can safely direct his attention to stimulating one of her nipples simultaneously either with a finger and thumb or orally.

I suppose the whole process of initiating him in this way may take ten days, or a fortnight. She will have to judge how slowly or how fast she can go. In the meantime, she should have been stepping up her own stimulation of him, stroking his back and his buttocks, fondling his penis and scrotum, caressing his inner thighs. By slow degrees she must show him what lovemaking is and how enjoyable it can be.

Some time in the third week *she* should stimulate her clitoris with his penis head. She can do this in two ways. She can ask him to lie on his side and she will lie on her side facing him; she will then reach down, take hold of his penis, and rub her clitoris with the head. Or she can get him to lie on his back, then kneel astride him with her back to him and her clitoral region between navel and penis tip. She then lifts his penis until it is upright, moves her clitoral area up to it, then either rubs against the penis or rolls it backwards and forwards over the clitoral area. I suggest she uses the first method first, as it is not so "daring."

By now I suggest she can put phase three into operation. This is to buy a good sex manual and leave it lying about so that he cannot miss it, if she feels it might be a mistake to give it to him directly with some such remark as, "I thought we might make our lovemaking more fun." I would like to think that my own book *Mainly For Wives* would be most helpful for two reasons—it is a book written for women, so that she could say she had come across it in a bookshop and thought it might help her to improve *her* lovemaking techniques; and also, though it is a book for women, it explains in clear straightforward language the lovemaking techniques a man can make use of. Unless he is a very odd young man he will want to read it, if only to see what some chap called Robert Chartham is putting women up to.

Well, that is the plan I put to Avis. Unfortunately a postal strike has intervened, and at the time of writing I have not heard from her how it has turned out.

Of course there are cases in which more direct approaches can be made. There are, for instance, some men who are such crashing bores sexually that one can afford to take them down a peg or two. Such men are always recognizable because they think of themselves as God's gift to women. The unhappy thing about it is that out of bed they are charming, kind, thoughtful, and fun, otherwise I doubt whether they would get any women to go to bed with them, let alone marry them. However, as soon as they begin to make love they become arrogant—they know what is best. Often they are not inept lovers, but unless their techniques do something for their partner, they might just as well be as ignorant as poor old David.

If the techniques such a man uses do not stimulate his partner as much as she would like to be and needs to be stimulated, she should not hesitate to tell him. He will be a bit shocked at first, but unless he is stupid as well as arrogant, he will admit the wisdom of her words and cooperate. He will quickly get over his shock, because in no time at all he will have convinced himself that he invented the new techniques. And what does it matter if he does, so long as both are happy and sexually satisfied?

The really expert lover, of course, never objects to being asked to caress and stimulate in certain ways, because he knows that there are almost as many different feminine preferences as there are women. For example, when a man stimulates the clitoris he nearly always does so directly. But for many women direct stimulation of the clitoris is not rousing at all, often the reverse; whereas running a fingertip up one side of the shaft and back again may be exquisite. Some women do not like the clitoral area to be touched at all, but like a finger, or two, to agitate the vagina entrance. Among women who do like direct clitoral stimulation some will only respond to very rapid light flicks of the fingertip, while others respond best to long, slow, heavy strokes.

No man, however expert he may be, can possibly be aware of these preferences, and goodness knows how many women are sexually unhappy and unsatisfied simply because they will not tell or show their partners what they would like to have done. If only they realized how grateful their partners would be for the opportunity to make themselves even better lovers than they already are, they would not hesitate for a moment.

There is rarely any need for a woman to be sexually frustrated because of her partner's faulty techniques, or techniques that do not do anything for her. There is need for a certain amount of intelligent guile to be used, but if the woman is at all experienced she should be able to sum up pretty well how to handle her problem. The main thing, in problems such as this, is to avoid wounding the partner's self-respect, and this is why the woman makes sure she understands his sexual character before taking him in hand. Of course, all this could be avoided if only couples were frank with one another from the start, and I am quite sure that most such difficulties will disappear once both women and men accept the fact that they have equal responsibilities when making love, to see that the partner is both satisfying and satisfied.

Chapter FOUR

"Is My Husband a Pervert?"

I think my readers would be as surprised as I constantly am by the number of times I am asked this question. What surprises me more than the question itself is the woman who asks it. Invariably she loves her husband dearly and sincerely, and is prepared to show her love for him in any way she can—almost in any way she can; she may have been married a few months, a year, three years, five or ten years; she has had experience of physical lovemaking and enjoys it; and she would be very happy to fall in with her husband's latest wishes, if only she could be assured by someone like me that what her husband is now wanting to do with her is not kinky. In 99 cases out of 100 there is not even a mild kinkiness involved, and in the odd case out, though there may be a suggestion of the bizarre, even then it is so faint a strangeness as to separate the activity by a million miles from true perversions.

Why, then, do women worry so about what they are sometimes asked to do during lovemaking?

I have an idea that it has to do in part with the basic difference that exists between the male and female responses to sexual stimulation; and in part to the conventions of feminine modesty and to the still widespread idea that sex is more for men than for women. The fact that the male responds to stimulation more quickly than a woman makes him more easily engage in sexual activity. The average man who is healthy and well-adjusted has few psychological hangups and is, therefore, extrovert to the extent that he does not hesitate to take the initiative in lovemaking. It follows that he is also more ready to experiment, provided he has the imagination. (Imagination, by the way, is a vital necessity in lovemaking. Though men are all that I have just said they are, unless

ADVICE TO WOMEN

they have sexual imagination they are dull lovers, and very quickly become lazy ones.)

Women, then, start at a disadvantage, but it is a disadvantage that is quickly overcome once the necessity for doing so has been taken to heart. The woman who has trained herself to be uninhibited in her sexual activities is without doubt a truly exciting lover. In fact, there are very few men who can surpass the really expert and imaginative woman. On the other hand, really uninhibited women are few and far between, and it seems to me that they will continue to be small in number until women in general realize, as I keep reminding them over and over again, that lovemaking is an *equal* partnership in which the woman has *equal* responsibilities with her lover for seeing that he obtains the highest degree of satisfaction and gratification, just as he is held responsible by her for providing her with the most intensely satisfying and gratifying experience that the circumstances of the lovemaking allow.

It is because women still hang on to the old idea that the man is the leader in sex that they retain the odd notion that there should be propriety in the bed; and not only propriety in the bed, but propriety of the bed, for many women are shocked by any suggestion that love should be made elsewhere—in the living room, the kitchen, the bath.

"My husband is sex-crazy," a woman writes to me. "Even when we're sitting watching the television he puts his hand up my skirt and wants to play with me. Of course, I won't let him, and I won't undo his fly and play with him either, as he asks me to do. How can I make him stop wanting to do this?"

"My husband is sex-crazy," another woman writes. "He wants to make love every other day. Sometimes it's every day. And another thing, he likes to spin it out as long as possible, though I like to get it over quickly. Is there anything he can take to make him more normal?"

"My husband is sex-crazy," exclaims another. "Every time he has a bath he wants me to join him and make love in the water. Surely this isn't natural?"

"My husband is sex-crazy," yet another protests. "He likes to watch me getting undressed. We go up to bed together, but he races and gets undressed quickly and jumps into bed, and his eyes never leave me as I take off my clothes. Do you think he's really a Peeping Tom?"

"My husband is sex-crazy," says another, but I don't

know whether she is protesting or reveling in her good fortune. "Ever since we've been married he has insisted on sleeping naked, and I went along with that because it seemed harmless. Now, though, he wanders about the house naked and I don't mind that either, but sometimes he does it when he's got an erection. He seems quite unperturbed about it, and I must say I find it very exciting, but what worries me is that he doesn't seem to have any modesty, and I'm beginning to wonder whether, as I say, he can't be a bit sex-crazy. I mean, surely a normal man wouldn't flaunt his erect penis, even in front of his wife."

The list of complaints (or comments, as I am sure they sometimes are) is so varied that I could fill up the entire space I have allotted to this chapter with it, and not once repeat myself. Most of them are of this harmless type, and are based on what the protestors believe to be affronts to their feminine modesty. And this is when I complain in return.

When the penis is put into the vagina, the two bodies assume the most intimate contact that two bodies can assume. If a woman can submit to having the most secret of her sexual recesses probed by her partner, how can she ever thereafter object that whatever her husband does to her or however he behaves before her is an affront to her modesty? It just doesn't make sense. Where lovemaking is used as a physical expression of emotional love how can there be any restraint? If there is restraint, then there cannot possibly be the *fullest* expression of love; and if there is not the fullest expression of love, to my mind there is little point in making love. Admit it freely that you take part in sexual intercourse not because you love your partner, but merely from lust—the desire to take part in sexual intercourse purely to experience the sexual sensations that you derive from it. Any woman who does engage in sexual activity for this reason certainly has abandoned every shred of modesty.

But where lovemaking is used as the expression of emotional love, there must be the fullest commitment of the two bodies to each other. The man's body is as much the woman's, as the woman's own body is to herself; and vice versa. This being so, she should be as familiar with it as she is with her own. When she is by herself, she would never dream of keeping her breasts and her genitals permanently covered. To bathe, she strips herself naked; to keep an eye on her figure, she stands naked before her mirror and surveys every curve. Since the man's body is equal to her own, ownership-wise, then she has every right to see it naked, in whatever state it is. Her private immodesty—for that is what she is displaying when she strips naked in private for whatever purpose—applies as much to her partner's body when they are alone together in the house.

The woman, then, who complains that her husband wanders about the house naked, even at times displaying his erect penis to her, and imagines she is justified in doing so on the grounds that her modesty is affronted, has no justification for her complaint at all. Surely she must realize that by complaining she is making one set of rules for herself, and another set for her husband. But when the marriage relationship is an equal partnership, how can this be? It makes a nonsense of the whole concept of equal partnership.

Not only that; by attempting to restrict her husband's naked activities she is actually trying to deprive herself of sexual experiences that can only make all the difference between a whole sexual relationship and a half sexual relationship. As I keep repeating over and over again, if the fullest love is to be expressed through lovemaking, then at each session of lovemaking each partner must aim at providing the other with the most intense orgasm sensations that the mood and circumstances of the occasion will allow. Every last degree of response must be coaxed out of each body. In order for this to happen both partners must administer and submit to every caress which will draw a response. Every caress on any and every part of the body!

Now, to be able to submit the whole body to every kind of caress requires the holding back of no part of the body from any caress. Put another way, to get the most out of lovemaking neither partner shall have what we call inhibitions. On the whole, women are much more sexually inhibited than men, chiefly, as I have explained above, because the man's sexual responses are much more direct, and equally because of the woman's sheltering behind false modesty. But men do have their sexual inhibitions, and one of the most common is the inability to let even their partners see them move about the room, or the house, naked with the penis erect. Most men do not mind their partners seeing their erections when they are laying down, but, strange though it may seem, many of these men are shy when it comes to walking about in the same state in the presence of their partners. I have an idea that what causes the shyness is the movement of the penis when the man moves, and, in some cases, if the erection is a very strong one, the slapping sound made by the penis during movement, as it hits against the belly. What is strange about this particular inhibition—at least I find it strange—is that since the man is so proud of his erection, assessing his virility and manhood by it, one would think he would be proud to let his partner, at all events, see it in all its glory, if only to impress upon her what a lucky woman she is to have a lover who has such a fine weapon. But the fact that the inhibition is fairly widespread is just another example of the male's illogicality in some sexual matters.

What I have been leading up to is this: The woman whose partner can and does display his erect penis has a partner who is wonderfully sexually uninhibited. Not long ago, a publisher who had invited me to discuss the possibility of my writing a book remarked early on in our conversation, "I wonder how long this boom in books on sex will last?" To which I replied, "Until a normal man can feel at ease walking down a busy street with an erect penis, and no one in the crowd takes any notice. Until that time comes sexual hangups will exist, and so long as there are sexual hangups there will be sexual problems, and a need for people like me." And I really believe this. The partner, therefore, who can freely display his erection is without doubt a man who has no sexual hangups, and a man without sexual hangups has the makings of a really expert lover.

Another difference between men and women lies in their responses to visual stimuli. A man can be very easily sexually roused by pictures of attractive naked women—not necessarily wholly erotic pictures—and by sculptures, and there are very few men indeed who do not respond with intense desire to the sight of a naked living woman. Very few women, on the other hand, are aroused by looking at pictures of naked men, no matter how handsome they are; and equally few are sexually moved by living naked men, with the possible exception that quite a number of women are aroused by the sight of the erect penis. The woman, therefore, whose partner likes to watch her undressing has a perfectly normal man for a lover, and she should be proud that she has the power to stimulate him sexually merely by undressing and appearing before him naked.

Equally proud, too, should be the woman whose partner is moved to fondle her, and want to be fondled by her, while watching the television. She should be flattered by the fact that her presence, fully clothed, and unprovocative, in surroundings that have no erotic features, should so attract her partner sexually that he wants to make love to her and for her to make love to him, then and there. Women whose husbands do react in this way and who make no objection, will admit, if asked, that they have nothing to complain about in their sex lives as a whole. One young husband I know now and again creeps up on his wife while she is washing up or is occupied at the kitchen table, fondles her until she is sexually roused, and then goes into her from behind.

"I'll admit," she told me, "that the first time he did it I was a bit taken aback, but I tried not to show it because I didn't want to hurt his feelings. Then as he made love to me I responded terrifically, and when I came my climax was so intense I nearly fainted. It happens like that every time. It doesn't take more than a few minutes, and usually we spend about an hour lovemaking when we're in bed. I think it must be because everything is so different from our usual lovemaking—the surroundings of the kitchen, standing up, and the position for coupling so different from the bedroom and the bed and so on. There's also the feeling, too, that we're being slightly naughty which adds to the excitement. I think if he did it often, it wouldn't be so good, but maybe it only happens once a month and I never know when it's going to happen."

Of course she is happy, because she has a sexually imaginative husband. Once more I say it—at the risk of being boring myself—but sexual boredom is the greatest enemy of sexual happiness. To avoid being sexually bored, the lovers must develop the widest possible range of loveplay techniques and use many different positions for coupling. The woman who complains that her husband wants to make love and couple in the bath (which can be one of the most exciting sexual experiences)—or standing up, or on a table or chair, or in front of a mirror, in the living room or the kitchen, anywhere, anyhow—far from complaining should be gratefully happy that she has such a sexually imaginative partner. She will never be sexually bored.

While on the subject of positions, the main complaint from women comes from those whose husbands want to use one of the rear-entry positions. Here again we come up against the woman's idea of feminine modesty, for the basis of the complaint—and very often for the refusal—is

"IS MY HUSBAND A PERVERT?"

the notion that if she submits to being entered from the rear she is being degraded, *because this is the position animals use*. But she is being made love to by a man who loves her and is trying to express his love for her through his lovemaking. Is such a man likely to do anything to degrade her? Of course not!

So we come to the cardinal rule: *Nothing that a couple can do to one another, or with one another, while making love can be degrading, depraved or morally wrong, always provided that neither partner is made to do something against his/her wishes and neither is physically or psychologically hurt by what they do.*

This applies equally to oral intercourse as to any other form of loveplay. It is, however, in connection with oral intercourse that women who complain about their husband's desire to use it employ the word *pervert*. "My husband wants me to let him suck my clitoris and play with my vulva with his tongue.* Surely the desire to do this must be perverted. I don't see how it can possibly be natural or normal." "My husband wants me to suck his penis† and gets quite upset when I refuse to. Have I married a pervert? It can't be normal to want that sort of thing. What can I do, because sometimes when I won't do it for him he refuses to make love to me?"

First of all, oral intercourse is absolutely normal and natural. (If you want to know why it is natural—though in speaking to women, I hesitate to explain—it is because all mammals at least do it instinctively, and if it is instinctive for other mammals, and, therefore, comes instinctively to them, it cannot be unnatural for humans if they have an instinctive need for it, too. How natural and instinctive it is for human beings is proved, in my view, by the fact that millions of people all over the world for thousands of years have been engaging in cunnilingus and fellatio. It has always been a popular form of loveplay in Southern Europe, and used to be so with us. The reason why it is something of a novelty to us—though every year thousands more people are incorporating it in their lovemaking—is because we are still suffering from the effects of the Victorian attitudes to sex.

The woman whose husband wishes to perform cunnilingus on her should not fear that by allowing him to do so she is being immoral, depraved, or perverted. As I said a

---

*The word for this is *cunnilingus*.

†The word for this is *fellatio*.

moment ago, if lovemaking is really and truly to be an expression of emotional love, both partners must see to it that they provide for each other the most intense physical experience possible. Stimulation of the clitoral area and vaginal entrance with lips and tongue provides a woman with the most voluptuous and sexually arousing sensations it is possible for her to have, with one possible exception—penis-vagina contact in the last phase of lovemaking when she has been taken over the point-of-no-return. It is illogical in the extreme that she should deprive herself of this experience on grounds of immodesty, abnormality, immorality, or whatever. Many pseudo-frigid women who cannot be brought to orgasm in any other way respond quite easily to cunnilingus. Are they to be deprived of sexual fullfillment on any grounds? If they are not—and they should not be—it is impossible to argue that anyone else should.

When women raise the red herring of perversion in connection with fellatio, they are not really concerned with questions of morals or deviations. Though they may be unconscious of it, it is really fear that is holding them back.

They are afraid that the Cowper's gland lubricating fluid, which most men produce when sexually roused, will taste. It does *not*; it is tasteless as well as being colorless and odorless. They are afraid, much more, that the partner will ejaculate in their mouths and that the semen will taste horrid, and that if they swallow it, it will do them physical harm.

First, though semen has a distinctive smell, its taste is what I call "light." That is to say, whatever taste it has is not unpleasant. Some say it has no taste at all—others that it tastes faintly of almonds; others that it has a somewhat sharp taste which produces a slightly burning sensation in the throat. In the latter case, this usually only happens if the partner has urinated shortly before making love. Very often it is not possible to tell when the semen has been ejaculated into the mouth, the reason being that when a man or a woman is sexually roused both produce an excessive amount of saliva which is the same temperature as the semen and which masks the flow of semen into the mouth. But in any case, whether one is conscious of it or not, it is not repulsive; only the idea of it may be.

As for being harmful, on the contrary it consists of many health-giving properties. Semen has three ingredients: (1) the sperm produced by the testicles, (2) the fluid produced by the seminal vesicles, and (3) the fluid produced by the prostate. Most of the volume comes from the seminal vesicles and it is this secretion which supplies the simple sugar-fructose which is essential for beginning and sustaining the motility of the sperm. Semen also contains very high concentrations of citric acid, vitamin C (ascorbic acid), and many enzymes, as well as bicarbonate and phosphate which protect the sperm from the action of the acids produced by the vaginal secretions. So there is nothing at all to do any harm.

However, if the woman still fears the effect of taking semen in her mouth, she can always come to an arrangement with her partner that he should warn her when he is about to come, so that she can withdraw. Mind you, the climax will not be the same for him, but the effects of oral stimulation before the point-of-no-return is reached are so very pleasant and exciting that most men are prepared to compromise in this way. Having made the promise, the man must keep it strictly. Otherwise the woman will be fully justified in refusing to perform fellatio on him again.

All women should know that many men develop a strong desire for fellatio—we call it a fellatio libido—which, if it is not satisfied, can lead to strong feelings of frustration, so strong, in fact, that they can throw the man's whole sexual functioning out of gear. The man in the letter I quoted obviously had such a strong fellatio libido, and by not satisfying it, his wife was heading for trouble. On the other hand, the man himself was very naughty in reacting as he did—refusing to make love to her. He was, in effect, trying to force her to do something which she did not want to do. By reacting in this way he was breaking the cardinal rule that neither partner must be forced to do something against his/her will. I must say, however, that her refusal even to try it was provocative in the extreme. If she really loved him, she would at least make an attempt to do what he wanted her to do. Only if she tried it, and still found it repulsive, could she justifiably claim that it was impossible for her; and I am quite certain that if she did try it and could not carry it through, he would be the first to absolve her. Many women have told me that though they had literally to force themselves to take the penis into the mouth, once they had tried it, they wondered what they had made all the fuss about.

Mind you, any man who wants his partner to fellate

him must, in duty bound, see to it that his penis is scrupulously clean. This applies very particularly to uncircumcised men. There really ought not to be any need for me to say this, because genital hygiene should be part and parcel of every man's general hygiene. Every man should wash his penis and scrotum twice a day—on washing in the morning and before going to bed, and every time before he makes love, at whatever time of the day. Englishmen, compared for instance with Frenchmen, are very lax in this respect, and I would say that any woman was fully justified in refusing to fellate a partner who did not wash himself thoroughly. Once he has washed, then there is far less danger to health from oral intercourse than there is in mouth-to-mouth kissing.

Fellation is not just a matter of putting the penis head in the mouth and sucking it. Of course this would give the man a good deal of pleasure, but as with any other loveplay technique, the aim must be to provide the highest degree of pleasure possible. To do this, again as with the sensitivity of the body as a whole, a knowledge of the sensitivity of the penis is a first consideration.

The skin covering the penis shaft is, of course, sensitive, but as a rule no more so than the skin anywhere else on the body not covering one of the recognized sensitive zones. The real site of sensitivity lies in the penis head, which, in fact, provides the man with the most sensitive of all his sensitive zones. In order to stimulate the penis head directly, if the man is uncircumcised it is essential that his foreskin is able to be slipped right back behind the rim which the head forms when it meets the shaft. (I have been told that the uncircumcised man whose foreskin does not slip back easily and whose penis head nerves cannot, therefore, be directly stimulated by the mouth or tongue, also finds the technique very exciting, and I have been taken to task for suggesting that unless these nerves are directly stimulated half the pleasure will be lost. Not being in a position to test this personally I asked a number of my friends who were uncircumcised to carry out a few experiments for me, first being fellated with the foreskin not drawn back, then with the foreskin drawn back, and to compare the two experiences sensation-wise. Though all testified that they thought the sensations were more intense with the foreskin back, I was really satisfied that the findings were conclusive, because if the foreskin has been retracted since boyhood, by the early twenties it will no longer completely cover the penis head when pulled for-

"IS MY HUSBAND A PERVERT?"

ward unless it is held forward. It cannot be held forward in the woman's mouth and this means that the very highly sensitive tip is exposed. Not only that, the foreskin slips back very easily and it is practically impossible for the woman to prevent it from doing so when her mouth is performing the movements of fellation. I mention all this, because whenever I express something in general terms, someone always writes to tell me that in his/her experience I am wrong. However, in this case I doubt very much whether I am, for it would be illogical to suggest that directly stimulated nerves do not respond more intensely than when stimulated through a layer of skin. I know that one swallow does not make a summer, but one man has written to me in support. He had an unretractable foreskin and was advised by his doctor to be circumcised. He had experienced fellation before the operation and afterwards, and claimed quite firmly, that there was no comparison—now that he is circumcised his sensations are many times more intense. Before leaving this point, I would like to set out my views on the fellation of a man whose foreskin will not draw back. In my view he should *not* be fellated for health reasons; if his foreskin has never been drawn back, it will be a seed-bed of many germs.)

As I said just now, the penis head is packed full of nerves and is the most sensitive part of the penis. But one can even be more precise than that. If your partner is not circumcised draw back the foreskin as far as it will go and, holding it back, look on the underside of the penis, and you will see that the ordinary skin of the shaft is joined to the special membrane covering the penis head by a little band of skin. This little band of skin is called the frenum, and it is absolutely jampacked with nerves. In most, though not all men, the frenum is the most sensitive area of the whole penis. Less than a quarter of an inch above the frenum is the opening of the urethra, the tube through which urine and semen pass out of the man. This short space and around the opening is also extremely well supplied with nerves, and this represents the second most sensitive area of the penis (though some men find it the most sensitive). The third most sensitive area is all round the edge of the rim which the penis head forms with the shaft and just under it. The rest of the head is moderately sensitive.

The nerves in the areas I have just described are sensitive to touch when the penis is soft and limp, and stimulation of them by mouth, tongue, or fingers will produce erection. When the penis is fully erect, the nerves become stretched and in that condition are much more sensitive than when the penis is limp. It is only on these areas that the woman should concentrate her oral caresses, especially the frenum, which responds to stroking with the tongue and sucking.

The penis head is, as I have said, very sensitive, not only to stimulation but to touch, and the woman applying oral caresses to it must be very careful all the time that she does not bite it or scratch it with her teeth. Quite a light bite or scratch can be so painful that the man will lose his erection immediately and may not be able to get it back that session. So the first technique of fellatio a woman must learn is to draw her lips down and under (or over) the edge of her teeth to avoid biting or scratching. At the same time, however, she should not draw her lips over her teeth rigidly tightly, but keep them as loose as possible.

In my view, the position adopted is important. Many men find it exciting to be fellated standing up, and for some unknown reason, when this happens, the woman nearly always kneels on the floor. Usually she has not thought to place a cushion to kneel on, and since, once started, she must continue—this seems to be a psychological urge—by the time she has finished her knees are very painful indeed. The position, however, is a good one, for the frenum is facing the woman and allows her to concentrate her tongue on it. Other men find that coming while standing is too exciting and leaves them feeling very weak and shaking at the knees, so that they have to sit down as soon as possible. These men find it more satisfactory to sit down while being fellated, with the woman again kneeling, again remembering to put down a cushion to kneel on. If the man prefers standing up, though, she will have to bend down, and it is really more comfortable for her if she sits on a chair. The really wise couple, however, will provide themselves with a stool of just the right height to bring her mouth level with the penis without having to bend her torso more than slightly.

Though I agree that there are occasions when it would be foolish not to continue fellation to orgasm, many couples find it more satisfying when used, not as an end in itself, but as a loveplay technique, the lovemaking finishing with penis-vagina contact. This is often acceptable to the woman who cannot overcome her objection to receiving the semen in her mouth. (By the way, there are very few men indeed who are not prepared to compromise with a partner and in return for her fellating them promise to withdraw before ejaculating. A woman should accept such a promise in good faith, because very often the fellatio libido that the man may have can be fully satisfied without his having to be fellated to orgasm. Realizing this, he will keep his promise. If, however, he breaks it, the woman will be fully justified in refusing to cooperate in this way again.)

If fellatio is used as a loveplay technique, then the best position is for the man to lie on the bed and the woman to recline beside him. When this position is adopted her face should be toward his face and her bottom toward his feet, rather than the other way round, because once again the frenum is brought directly under her tongue, which does not happen if she has her bottom toward his face and her face toward his feet.

Most couples who have adopted oral intercourse agree that simultaneous oral caresses are exciting only just short of the excitement provided by penis-vagina contact. In order to carry out this simultaneous stimulation, one or other variants of the position known as "69" has to be used. One variant is for the couple to lie side by side with their faces within easy reach of each other's genital areas. It is a very restful position, but it has the drawback that the man is not very well placed to caress the clitoris and vaginal area.

By far the most satisfactory "69" position is when the man lies on his back and the woman crouches astride and above him. Her genital area will be over his face, and her own mouth is within easy reach of his penis.

The techniques of applying fellatio are not complicated, but it is surprising how many women lack the imagination to think them out for themselves. As I remarked earlier, fellatio does not consist merely of the woman enclosing the penis head in her mouth and sucking on it. She should begin with kissing the penis all over, and particularly the tip, which is very responsive to the lips. This can be followed by a number of varieties of caress, for example, running the tongue round the edge of the rim, the tip of the tongue round under the rim, licking the frenum and tip of the penis with the tongue and *very, very* lightly nipping the frenum between the lip-covered teeth. Blowing on the penis head and under the rim is also very exciting.

When the penis is at last taken into the mouth, as much of it should be taken in as you can manage without retching. At the same time as you suck move the mouth up and down on the penis. Most men like to control these movements, so if your partner puts his hands on your head to do this—obviously he cannot do this in one of the "69" positions—go with the rhythm his hands make.

You will have to hold his penis away from his belly, if he is lying down, and while you are doing so, you should move this hand up and down that part of the penis which does not go into your mouth. With your other hand fondle his testicles, again *very, very* lightly as they are very tender, and if you press too hard you will hurt him intensely and he will lose his erection.

If his testicles are not too large, as a variation take them into your mouth and suck them. Most men find this very arousing, but again take good care not to nip them with your teeth or suck on them too hard.

As his sensations increase you will notice that his testicles will now and again move up toward the base of his penis—inside the scrotum—pause for a second or two and then lower themselves again. When he is approaching the point-of-no-return he will begin to breathe heavily and he will automatically push up and lower his pelvis rhythmically. At the same time, his testicles will ascend more frequently, pause longer in the higher positions, and not descend quite so low as they did previously. When this begins to happen you will know that he will ejaculate within thirty to sixty seconds. If you cannot take his semen in your mouth and withdraw, you must continue to stimulate his penis with your hand, using rapid movements, until he comes. If you do not do this, though he may ejaculate, he will have only half an orgasm which will leave him very frustrated.

As I think I have shown, oral intercourse in an art, like all other lovemaking techniques. It cannot fail to provide both partners with extremely pleasant sensations, and improve the intensity of the orgasm, whether it is prolonged to the end or used only as a loveplay technique. It is worth any time and patience making oneself really proficient at it.

So please get out of your head that it is neither natural nor normal. It is not a perversion for a man (or a woman) to desire it.

There are very few perverted husbands around. I ask you to believe this, if you still have any lingering doubts. Let me repeat the great cardinal rule of lovemaking:

There is nothing which a man and woman can do together sexually in the privacy of their homes, which is immoral or depraved, *provided both get enjoyment out of it, and neither is forced by the other to do something against his/her wishes.*

Chapter FIVE

What is Sexual Excess?

Dear Mr. Chartham: I am rather worried because my husband seems always wanting to make love. We have been married for sixteen months. I am twenty-five and my husband is twenty-seven. We did not actually make love before we married, but during our courting days I had an idea that my boyfriend, as he was then, was quite passionate by the way he kissed and caressed me. I didn't mind it. To be quite honest, it was one of the exciting things I found about him.

In the few months after we married, we made love almost every day. This didn't worry me either, because in the excitement of being married to the man I loved, I was quite ready to be made love to whenever he wanted to. I knew, though, that this wasn't the real sexual me, because from the time I first became aware of having any sexual desire, I don't suppose I felt the need to masturbate more than half a dozen times a year, and being sexually roused five or six times a week was, I was sure, my way of reacting to the new, wonderful experience of being married. Mind you, I had expected to have an increase in desire, but not to this extent.

I thought at first that my husband was reacting to this new experience in the same way, and that, in time, he would, so to say, get the novelty out of his system and settle down sexually. This hasn't happened. Well, I suppose it has to a small extent, because we make love on an average five times a week, while in the early days it was often seven, and never less than six.

Don't you think making love so often is not good for a man who has quite a heavy and responsible job? How often ought we to make love? I don't mean a set round figure per week, but a weekly average.

Please don't think I find it irksome or tiring. There

WHAT IS SEXUAL EXCESS? 63

are some times when I wish he wouldn't, but I never refuse him. He is such a skillful lover that he always rouses me, and I find it quite nice even though sometimes I don't come. It's really him I'm worried about.

What is sexual excess? This is a question I am often asked, and it is a question that is impossible to answer, because individually we differ so much and even from occasion to occasion in the same individual, that what may be regarded as excessive for some is normal for others, and vice versa.

How often we want to make love is all bound up with what is known as our sex drive, and this is also one of the most misunderstood of the many misunderstood aspects of sex. Let me try to explain about the sex drive.

The sex drive is our response to certain chemical reactions that are always taking place within our bodies. This chemistry makes itself known to us physically by certain sensations which we experience from time to time, and these sensations build up eventually until our sex organs prepare themselves for intercourse—the erection of the penis in the man, and the erection of the nipples and clitoris and the swelling of the vaginal lips in the woman.

The first sign that our sex drive is beginning to work is a sensation of being "on edge." This sensation is felt in the penis, scrotum, thighs, and lower belly of the man; in the vagina, clitoral area, breasts, thighs, and lower belly in the woman. It may be felt only occasionally at first; we may be aware of it only for a moment or two, then something distracts our attention from it. By degrees, however, it builds up until we feel a definite physical sensation which spreads from the sexual organs to the general nervous system. When this stage is reached, we know that the tension will only be relieved by sexual activity which will result in orgasm.

When we come, it is as if we were emptying certain of our organs which felt as though they had become swollen to the bursting point. This does actually happen to the man. His seminal vesicles become so full that they can hold no more, and send their fluid plus sperm down to the prostate, where they join with the prostate fluids, thus forming semen, which is spurted out of the penis as the man comes.

This emptying process is not quite so obvious in the woman. She does not ejaculate any fluid when she comes, but the actions of certain muscles which come into play at her climax relax the taut sexual nerves which have made her aware of her sexual needs.

The sex drive, which is born in all of us, is the result of the interaction of various glands. Among these glands in the man are the testicles and the pituitary, the latter being a gland about the size of a large pea, situated in a small pocket of the bony floor of the skull in the center of the head at the top of the spine; the corresponding woman's glands are the ovaries and the pituitary.

The function of the pituitary gland is to stimulate the production of hormones, which are chemical substances produced by the glands and passed directly into the blood. The various sets of glands in our bodies produce quite a variety of hormones which affect our physical development and behavior in one way or another. The sex glands produce sex hormones under the direction of the pituitary gland.

The male sex hormones are called androgens, the best known being testosterone, which is made by the testicles. The chief female sex hormones are estrogen and progesterone, which are made by the ovaries.

Testosterone and estrogen are responsible for our sex drive. Progesterone develops the woman's breasts at puberty and thereafter prepares the womb to receive the fertilized egg.

Another hormone found in both men and women is Prolan A or FSH (follicle-stimulating hormone). In women it matures the egg nestling in its follicle in the ovaries; in men, it stimulates the production of sperm by the testicles.

As I said earlier, the strength of the sex drive varies from individual to individual, and from occasion to occasion in the same individual. Put another way, there are some men and women who are far more sexually active than others, and some who are sexually less demanding than others. In fact, there is scarcely an individual whose sex drive is exactly as strong as another's.

Broadly speaking, however, there are three main groups of men and women distinguishable by their sex drive and, consequently, by their sexual activity. First, a comparatively small group of what we term *high-sexed* (or highly passionate) men and women. At the other extreme is another group, not quite so small as the first, who experience sexual tension only infrequently. We call them *low-sexed*.

WHAT IS SEXUAL EXCESS?

In between is a very large group termed the *average-sexed*. Since there are very many more average-sexed than there are high-sexed and low-sexed, we take them to represent the norm. They may roughly be said to experience sexual desire, arousal, and the need for orgasm two or three times a week (in their twenties slightly more often). The low-sexed may experience sexual desire, arousal, and the need to come only once every two weeks or once a month. The high-sexed, on the other hand, have at least a daily urge, and often a twice-daily or thrice-daily urge. These frequencies are the average figures for all three groups for the ages between seventeen and thirty-five. As we grow older, our sex drive becomes less strong.

There are, then, men and women whose sex drives are far more powerful and more demanding than are the sex drives of others. Those who have a powerful sex drive have to have relief from the tensions it builds up more frequently than those with a less powerful sex drive.

What we have to accept is that there is no way in which a man or woman can regulate his/her sex drive. Though a low production of a certain hormone can be boosted by injections of this particular hormone, *there is no method by which hormone production can be cut down*. Since, for various reasons which I need not go into here, hormone injections are only given in the most extreme cases—say, of a man whose sex drive has almost disappeared altogether—by and large, we have to accustom ourselves to the fact that we are landed with our sex drive; and even more important, so are our partners with theirs. In our physical sex life, our sex drive controls our sexual needs. There is no getting away from it.

Ideally, of course, a man or woman should marry a partner with a similar sex drive, but love does not always, in any practical sense, take the strength of the sex drive into account. Even if a couple were absolutely frank with one another and discussed their sex needs before they got engaged, I doubt very much whether it would make any difference to their decision to marry, or even consider if they ought to. But if they find that one partner's sexual needs are greater than the other's, they ought certainly to try to find some means of closing the gap.

Since there are many many more average-sexed men and women than either high-sexed or low-sexed, more often than not there is no great problem of inequality of sex drive. On the other hand, if my mail is anything to go by, the problem does crop up more often than one would expect it to.

In many cases there is probably no problem at all. The girl whose letter I quoted at the beginning of this chapter only thought she had a problem, because she imagined her husband might be doing himself some physical harm by the frequency of his lovemaking. She showed, nevertheless, that though they had differing sex drives the differences could be removed by cooperation.

And cooperation is the solution—and understanding of what is happening!

If these two faculties exist, then I honestly do not think any problem need arise, for the simple reason that neither men nor women, high-sexed, average-sexed or low-sexed, can *only* become sexually aroused in response to their sex drives. I am sure that it is in the experience of all couples who have regular opportunities for lovemaking that now and again they go to bed without any intention of or any desire to make love. Then something happens. The man may put his hand over a breast as he snuggles down beside his partner; his pubic hair may brush lightly against her buttocks; or he may kiss the nape of her neck; or the woman, scarcely realizing what she is doing, as she snuggles up to him, may reach down and take his quiet penis in her hand; her nipples may brush against his arm; or she suddenly becomes aware of his sexy smell—and hey presto! the blood is rushing into penis, nipple, clitoris, and vaginal lips, and before they know where they are they are making love and loving it.

I have been gathering a few figures about this for some time now, and it seems pretty certain that most ordinary couples up to the age of forty-five, at any rate, make love twice deliberately, i.e., not in response to their sex drives, to every three times that they do respond to their sex drives. This is particularly so of men and women who do honestly use their lovemaking to express their love for one another. Love does not wait upon the sex drive, and out of the sheer happiness of loving, or because one or other of the partners wants to say "thank you" for some special or unexpected consideration, there are frequent occasions when the couple turn to lovemaking to do just that.

Mind you, I think probably that it might not happen so often as it does were it not for the fact that normal healthy men in all these sex drive categories, even when they are *not* responding to their sex drives, can be sexually roused, have a very strong erection, and come, all in the

WHAT IS SEXUAL EXCESS?

space of two to five minutes. If the penis did not spring to attention quite so readily, maybe there would be less "deliberate" lovemaking than there is, but since the results are just as satisfying and pleasant as when one is responding to the sex drive, I don't see any point in trying to differentiate.

There is another thing, too, which is widely overlooked in this connection. Though the woman may not respond to stimulation so quickly as the man does, even if she has a definite desire not to make love, she can always be roused if her partner is a skillful lover to the extent of accepting penis-vagina contact, and if she loves her partner and he loves her, can end up by enjoying it and being sexually satisfied.

It is my experience that where a woman complains of the frequency of her husband's lovemaking—even when he is high-sexed and she is not—she does not find lovemaking a chore because she is not responding to her sex drive but for some other reason. Prominent among such reasons (which may not always be consciously recognized by the woman) is fear of an unwanted pregnancy and the quite mistaken notion that by making love so often her husband is "using" her for his selfish ends, and she is making herself "cheap" by submitting to every sexual approach he makes. The fear of pregnancy can be overcome by the simple method of seeking expert contraceptive advice and heeding it. The second reason is a whole lot of poppycock, and any woman who shelters behind it cannot *really* love her partner.

Of course, I can understand the woman who has difficulty in reaching orgasm finding frequent lovemaking a bit irksome, but as I have tried to explain in Chapter 2, very often the nonachievement of orgasm is the result of faulty techniques on the part of the man—or of both—or of a lack of communication between them. But even so, women who really love their husbands do not complain, and though they may only come in one out of five sessions of lovemaking, are happy on the other four occasions simply because they have made their husbands happy.

Another point that is misunderstood by women—and many men, as well—is the old excuse of tiredness. I don't know how many letters I have in my files like these:

> Dear Mr. Chartham: Please help me. I am thirty-two and the mother of three wonderful children aged seven, five, and four. We have been married nine

years, and my husband is a fine husband and father. We are not badly off, but I cannot get help for more than two hours a week, and consequently I have to do most of the housework myself. If you have any children of your own, you will know what a lot of work they make, but I am not complaining about that. I don't mind how hard I work to keep them and my husband happy and well. But what my husband does not seem to understand is how tired I get.

There are some days when I feel I could fall asleep on my feet while washing up the supper things, and when we go to bed, all I want to do is curl up and sleep. But my husband wants to make love, three, sometimes four, times a week, and he just can't get it into his head that very often I'm much too tired to respond to him. He doesn't like it when I sometimes turn away from him, and he gets annoyed, even angry. Could you possibly write to him and tell him that when a woman is tired, the last thing she wants to do is to make love? . . .

Dear Dr. Chartham: I am getting very frustrated. We have been married fifteen years and have teenage boy twins. I am forty-six and my husband is forty-seven. During the first ten years of our married lives, our sex was perfect. We often made love, sometimes two or three times at the weekends even though we may have done so three times during the week. Now we are lucky if we make love once a week. I admit I don't want to make love now quite so often as I did three or four years ago, but I certainly want to more than once a week. To get my relief I have to masturbate, which I do at least twice, more often three times a week. And what's the reason? My husband is too tired!

I know he works very hard and has a very responsible job, and he also does quite a lot of voluntary work for one of the local political parties. The first thing he says when he comes home every evening, after he's said hello to us, that is, "God, I'm weary!" And I know what that means! No lovemaking tonight! When we go to bed, he's always in bed before I've taken off my face, and quite often by the time I get into bed, he's asleep or pretending to be. On the occasions when I try to start lovemaking, he nearly always says, "Not tonight, dear, I'm tired!" It's driving me crazy, honestly, Dr. Chartham. In my crazier moments I think I shall have to take a lover. I'm not so sure that it is such a crazy idea. Can you suggest anything I can do?

Both the writer of the first letter and the husband in the second letter—he is really a "lazy" husband, and I shall be dealing with him in the next chapter in more detail—are making their tiredness an excuse for not making love, and they are justifying their excuse by convincing themselves that because they are tired they *cannot*—and should not be expected to—make love. Much of this tiredness is actually a state of mind. Except in extreme cases of mental or physical exhaustion—and they must be *extreme* cases—the body and mind are quite capable of responding sexually.

In fact, I go much further. To make love when one is tired is not only possible, it is also beneficial. I work quite hard myself, beginning my day, six days a week, at 4 to 4:30 A.M. and writing solidly or seeing people until the TV news at 6 P.M. when I stop, even if I'm in the middle of a sentence. Sometimes I am pressed by a publisher with an eye on a delivery date, and then I do occasionally carry on after supper to 11 P.M. That means that I have worked fifteen or sixteen hours a day, and I may have to do this for two or three days on end. So I know what physical and mental exhaustion is. But it is at these times that I find lovemaking is what keeps me going. I get into bed so weary I don't know how to lie comfortably, so mentally tired that I can scarcely think, and my nerves so taut it would seem that the slightest jar will snap them. Then I am made love to, and as hands pass over me, and the sensations of arousal mount, all the tautness and the tiredness begins to retreat. When eventually the climax sweeps over me, I feel at once relaxed, mentally and physically, and we snuggle down and sleep. Four hours later, I am awake and fresh, ready for another day. And I am over sixty!

The whole process of arousal seems to gather up all the jangled nerves that spring from tired limbs and tired minds. As the sensations mount they take over the body, displacing all other sensations, especially the unpleasant ones. The explosion of orgasm, even when not intense, must by the very nature of what happens in our bodies as it occurs, release nerves from the strain they are under and put to flight all thoughts but those of pleasure, gratitude, and love.

If, then, it is beneficial to make love when one is weary, there is little likelihood of being able to make love to excess or to harm oneself by frequent lovemaking. This latter, in respect of men, is a leftover of a wrong idea our Victorian ancestors had about the nature of semen. They believed that if semen was not ejaculated, it passed into the bloodstream and enriched the blood and so contributed to the health of the man. We know now that semen not only does not, but cannot, enter the bloodstream under any circumstances nor will the rich ingredients it contains benefit the body in any way if it is retained.

One day, I know, you will get tired of my repeating that we all react to sex in our own individual ways and that there are tremendous differences in our needs and responses. I know of two cases of young men of the same age which illustrates this. They are both twenty-two, and the first responds to his sex drive with masturbation roughly once every ten days, while the other masturbates to orgasm four times a day. Recently the second underwent a test under laboratory conditions, and in one hour he masturbated himself to orgasm thirteen times. He suffered no ill effects and when asked forty-eight hours later how many orgasms he had had since the test, reported nine. He was not an obsessive masturbator, but a normal and healthy young man physically and psychologically merely responding to a high sex drive.

If any guide can be given, then, as to what is not excessive sexual activity, I think it can only be this: If you respond always to your sex drive and make love deliberately two or three times in addition, you won't go wrong. If you do overdo it a bit—and there can be occasions when this may happen—you will soon know. You will develop an ache in the groin and a dull nagging pain in the small of your back. Should these symptoms occur, lay off all sexual activity for twenty-four hours and you will be as right as rain again.

Chapter SIX

The Lazy Husband

I feel certain that it may surprise many people to know that I am constantly getting letters from women complaining that their husbands do not make love to them often enough. Usually the complaint is just the reverse—that the husband wants to make love too often. I was a bit taken aback when I first began to receive these letters, and then it began to occur to me that there are sexually lazy husbands—far too many, in fact, if my figures are correct.

Dear Mr. Chartham: I have a problem and I wonder if you could help me with it, please. I am twenty-five and my husband is twenty-seven. I have one baby and am five months' pregnant. My problem is that I can't rouse my husband.

When we first married it was all right, because I managed to get him aroused fairly easily. Lately, however, nothing I do seems to have any effect. I have read your two books *Mainly For Wives* and *Sex For Advanced Lovers* and tried all the arousal methods you mention, to the best of my ability, but nothing seems of any avail. He has never been a man to show his feelings very much, but now there is just no response.

It makes me feel very inadequate, because my husband can arouse me very easily, when he tries, which isn't very often now, and only happens when I ask him to make love to me, which I don't like to do very often because it makes me feel rather cheap. I have never heard of any other woman having to ask her husband to make love to her. I am beginning to wonder if there is something wrong with me, as I can't get him roused. Whenever I try to take the initiative in making love, I never seem to get the movement right and I land up hurting him.

You say in your books that the tip of the penis is

supposed to be very sensitive to touch, but when I touch my husband's penis, it hurts him. He is not circumcised, but this surely should make no difference?

I would be very grateful for any suggestions you can make and look forward to hearing from you at your earliest convenience.

When I studied this letter, it seemed to me that it contained three key phrases—(1) "When we first married it was all right, because I managed to get him aroused fairly easily . . ." (2) ". . . my husband can arouse me very easily when he tries [but this] only happens when I ask him to make love to me," and (3) "He is not circumcised." The first and second phrases indicated, I thought, that here was a young man of twenty-seven—probably low-sexed, and certainly less high-sexed than his wife—who was only infrequently roused by his sex drive but was too lazy, too inconsiderate, to take his wife's greater sexual needs into account and put himself out just a little bit to see that her needs were satisfied.

In fact, this is a variation of the classic case in the category of sex problems. A young man with a low sex drive quite naturally wants to marry, and he eventually finds a girl with whom he feels he can settle down comfortably. During the first months of marriage—perhaps for the first year—the novelty of lovemaking induces him to rouse himself sexually more often than he would be prompted to do by his sex drive. Maybe, too, he senses his wife's higher sex drive and unconsciously accepts it as a challenge. In so doing, he unfortunately misleads his wife about his true sexuality.

As the novelty wears off, he makes love less and less frequently, responding, probably, only when his sex drive prompts him to. In fact, he finds lovemaking except to relieve tension a bit of a chore, and he takes refuge behind his sex drive. Clearly his wife is puzzled by this new state of affairs. In the initial period, he has made love to her sufficiently frequently for her not to suspect that his sex drive is less strong than hers, and she begins to worry now (a) whether something physically is wrong with him or (b) whether there is something wrong with her. Her own sex drive is as strong as ever it was, but he seems not to notice, and to arouse his interest, without actually having to ask him to make love to her, she makes love to him, and to her dismay, she finds him unresponsive.

THE LAZY HUSBAND

Most men—and women—with low sex drives, understandably perhaps, do not have the same interest in sex that average-sexed men have. They rarely study photographs of the pinup variety, or seek out books with sexual themes in order to be titillated; and they are apt to find their companions' sex conversation and display of interest in sex rather revolting. Only very, very rarely do they show even an interest in lovemaking techniques, and I have not yet met a low-sexed man who has read a sex manual or tried to discover what makes him and his partner tick sexually.

The low-sexed are predisposed to be sexually lazy, because they are not so often prompted by their sexual natures to engage in lovemaking. Yet when they do make love they are as satisfied by the experience as any man is who makes love many times more frequently. They are also quite capable of being roused as easily as any other man by direct stimulation of the penis at times when the sex drive is not operating, but only if they enter into the spirit of it and are not taking refuge in being lazy. Some low-sexed men have tried to argue with me that they find making love at times when the sex drive is not operating unpleasant. Such an argument shows that they do not use their lovemaking at any time to express their emotional love for their partner.

By compromise on the part of both, it is perfectly possible for an average-sexed woman married to a low-sexed man to have a really satisfactory sex life. It will mean that he will be a little more sexually active than he would be if he responded only to his sex drive, while she will have to be content to obtain some of her relief from masturbation, or from heavy petting by her husband if he really does not feel like full intercourse (and he should be prepared to help her in this way always).

But if the man is not prepared to compromise and his wife tries to entice him into activity, there is always a great risk of his responses being seriously affected by a psychological reaction. What causes it is this. The woman's frequent attempts to get her husband to respond sooner or later bring home to him the fact that he has a lower sex drive than she has. Now, although he may be low-sexed, he still holds the same view of the male's role in sex—that he is the sexual initiator who must dominate his partner sexually—as most other men hold. He realizes that his sexual needs are less than his partner's and this makes him feel sexually inferior.

The psychiatrists refer to these feelings of inferiority as feelings of sexual *inadequacy,* and sexual inadequacy can affect a man in several ways. In the first place it creates a vicious circle; his fear of being inadequate makes him inadequate. Physically the inadequacy reveals itself in two ways; either the man responds to stimulation and has a normal erection, but ejaculates too soon, before his partner has had time to come herself—or he does not respond to stimulation at all, in other words, becomes impotent. In many cases, though the realization of inadequacy affects the man psychologically in the first place, this primary psychological cause is replaced by another more subtle and more dangerous one—he refuses (generally unconsciously) to respond to his wife's stimulation *to punish her for being more sexually adequate than he is.*

I would very much have liked to talk with both the letter-writer and her husband, but they lived very far away. I wanted to do so because I had a feeling that it was feelings of sexual inadequacy that were at the root of the wife's inability to rouse her husband. I suggested that the next time I was in the area we might arrange to meet, but this he flatly refused to do, and because of this refusal I feared that he was intent (though again perhaps unconsciously) on punishing the wife because she was sexually superior.

For the point is this: In my experience if one can reach a man suffering from feelings of inadequacy before the desire to punish sets in, a simple straightforward chat can usually convince him that he need *not* be inadequate if he will compromise with his partner in the ways I have suggested. On the other hand, after the desire to punish has set in, only a long course of psychotherapy is indicated to remove the psychological block, and it may not be successful.

The third key phrase interested me—"He is not circumcised"—because I believed that this, too, might be a further indication of the husband's state of mind. The wife did not say in her letter whether the foreskin could be pulled, easily, right back behind the rim. In some cases when it will not, an inexpert handling of the penis which tries to pull the foreskin back will hurt considerably. Alternatively, if the foreskin would pull right back easily, the pain—psychologically caused—could be another attempt by the husband to reject his wife's stimulation. The pain could be absolutely genuine, but it would cease as soon as the husband came to terms with his state of mind.

Actually, in this case, the foreskin did slip back easily.

There is very little one can do by letter to help cases of this sort. In fact, there is little one can do at all if the husband will not cooperate. All I could suggest was that the wife insist on having a frank talk with her husband to try to discover what was really wrong from his point of view. If he would not cooperate, even in this, then she was faced with two alternatives, one of which in her condition she could not possibly accept: either she should satisfy her sexual needs by self-stimulation, or seek a divorce and make a new start.

> Dear Mr. Chartham: I would be very pleased if you could help me with my problems. I am twenty-three years of age, and just married for three months. Firstly, my husband wants intercourse about every night, but does nothing to arouse me, but makes me excite him by handling his penis, and frequently when doing this, he comes, but I have to continue till he has another erection, when he wants intercourse. I never reach a climax before he is finished, when he goes to sleep leaving me aroused but far from satisfied.
>
> Secondly, he has what I would call a very large penis (not having seen other males) being about seven inches long and very thick. My problem is that when erect, and he forces it into me, it is just painful, and I cannot enjoy sex, as my vagina is far too tight for a penis of this size. I have told him about this, but he says it is nonsense as all vaginas will stretch to take penises of any size.
>
> I would appreciate your help as I just cannot enjoy sex like this.

It is not just the low-sexed man who becomes the lazy husband. This second man is high-sexed, but he is not only a lazy husband, he is also an inconsiderate, selfish, sexual boor. It is rare to find a sexual boor among the highsexed, because they are usually sensitive people, who enjoy their uninhibited sexual activity, and want their partners to have as much pleasure as they do, being prepared to go to any lengths to see that they do. One finds this type of husband more among the average-sexed, and I'm afraid they constitute one of the most numerous classes of sex-lazy husbands.

As a rule they are conceited men, and are selfish in

other aspects of living besides sex. All they are concerned with is their own sexual pleasure and satisfaction. They regard their partners as sexual chattels, there merely to provide them with their own gratification.

There is only one way in which a woman married to such a man can react. She must go on strike, making him understand quite forcibly that she will stay out until he agrees to make love to her and arouse her and see to it that she gets as much relief from her tensions as he does from his. If he has no knowledge of loveplay techniques she must get him a good book on the subject and make him read it and put its advice into practice, after first having read it herself, so she may know what he ought to be doing. She can encourage him to take this course by offering to improve her own techniques of making love to him, and undertaking to participate in any sexual activity he may suggest that is not totally out of the question for her to accept.

While his penis is somewhat larger than average, if her descriptions of its dimensions are correct, he is quite right in saying that any vagina can stretch to accommodate it. But so that it does not hurt her, until regular intercourse has permanently stretched her vagina, the penis must be well lubricated before he tries to put it in. It is another sign both of his selfishness and laziness that he does not use a lubricant of some sort. If he was not lazy he would buy one of the recommmended lubricants that are easily obtainable; but there is no need even for him to exert himself that much. One of the best lubricants there is, is saliva. It costs nothing, it is always in good supply, because when both men and women are sexually aroused their production of saliva more than doubles, and it is easily transferred from the mouth to the penis by the fingers. If he refuses to do this himself, she must insist on doing it before she lets his penis anywhere near her vagina.

Unless he is absolutely thick-skinned, I think her threat to go on strike will bring him to his senses. If it does not she must seriously think of her future, because unless she breaks him in now, she will never have a happy sex life with him.

When the sex-lazy husband is young, he may be lazy because he is ignorant. There is no need for any woman to put up with this, because if she sets about it in the right way she will nearly always find he is willing to learn. In fact, they can have a good deal of fun learning together, because he has as much right to be made love to expertly as she has. But the minimum a woman should demand—even when she has to accept the fact that her lover is not sexually imaginative or daring—is arousal to the threshold of the point-of-no-return before she accepts the penis; and if she does not come during coupling, she must insist that he brings her to orgasm manually or orally when they are uncoupled. This, I repeat, is the *minimum* demand she should make on him.

There are sex-lazy husbands of all ages, and the husband in his forties who can't be bothered sexually is usually the man who is intent on his career, who devotes all his energies to his job, and uses his physical tiredness as an excuse not to make love. I referred to him in the last chapter.

No wife should put up with such a husband. If she does, she is storing up for herself a crabbed, unsatisfactory old age. Her main weapon against such a husband is the proven fact that the sexual apparatus must have regular exercise if it is to continue to function. Not long ago, it was the theory that of all the parts of the body, the sexual parts alone did not require exercise to keep them toned up. We know now that this is not true. As a result of their investigations, Masters and Johnson, the famous American sexual researchers, have shown that the earlier men and women begin their sexual activities and the more often they make love, the later in life they will be capable of making love.

"Are you intending to be a dropout from sex now?" the wife of the forties and fifties sex-lazy husband should ask him. "Because if you are, then I am going to look around for another partner. Once you've become a dropout from sex, you remain a dropout for the rest of your life, and that does not appeal to me."

It may take a good deal of patience and effort to make such a sex-lazy husband snap out of his laziness, but if you really value your happiness as a senior citizen, you must make him see sense. He will be so much better for it, in any case. His work will be more inspired, and he will achieve his ambitions so much more easily if he is a whole person—and no one can be a whole person if they have no sex life.

Probably the largest class of sex-lazy husbands is to be found among the late fifties and early sixties.

ADVICE TO WOMEN

Dear Mr. Chartham: I feel I am probably imposing on your good nature by writing to you, but since reading your book *Sex and the Over-50s,* I am encouraged to ask your advice. Arising from this you will realize that my husband and I have a problem though to each of us it appears different.

My age is fifty and for some years before I took on my present full-time job as a probation officer, I did a good deal of voluntary social work. My husband is sixty-three, a retired accountant, who now works a couple of days a week keeping the books for his golf club. The framework of our lives is a happy and interesting one and it would grieve us both deeply if this were disrupted by separation. That I have even contemplated this course would shock my husband, and will give you some indication of my distress.

I have used all endeavors to make our marriage relationship a rich one, but over the years my husband's sexual need of me has diminished. I in turn have tried to be patient and loving, my only relief from tension being found in tears. These I conceal from my family (a married son and a married daughter) and from my husband when I can, as I know from experience that he does not know what I am wanting. He is a kind man and tries to compensate for what he calls his inadequacies by being helpful round the house, and, finances permitting, providing me with anything I want; in other words "keep her happy at any price, ignore the problem, and perhaps it will go away."

Some six or seven years ago I suffered acute depression but this was promptly dealt with by my understanding doctors; however, this, together with the menopause, has provided a useful excuse when I am not my usual happy smiling self. Twice recently I have tried to talk to my husband about our situation (me in tears, and he feeling humiliated and helpless) but the answer is that he was never strongly sexed and that I married the wrong man. This I can't accept, as I still love him dearly and I know his world centers around me.

After a "to-do" on my part he begins to respond even to the extent of infrequent intercourse, but as soon as I appear happy and content he relaxes his efforts and we are back to the old platonic relationship. The description you give in your book on pages 97 and 98 seems to fit me exactly.

I do indeed feel radiant, and though it is possibly illogical I feel deeply hurt that my husband does not find me attractive. To take a lover would be an answer, but I am still romantic enough to want love with a sexual relationship—this also at the moment rules out masturbation. I am really feeling too tired to go on trying and in admitting defeat I am left hopeless.

Several times over the years my husband has promised to consult his doctor about his impotence, but has never done so. Some six years ago he had a prostatectomy but to our mutual surprise he was afterwards able to achieve an erection and we had normal intercourse, so I do not understand him when he says it is physically impossible for him to make love to me now. He will *not* discuss his feelings, but lapses into hurt, stony silence.

We are known and envied locally as being the ideal married couple, but I do not think I can continue with this double act. Neither can I put myself through the nightly torture of sharing a double bed (though a couple of seconds help here). However to sleep apart would, I know, wreak immeasurable damage to a teetering structure, and my husband would be unbearably hurt. So much so, that the future would be a downward trend away from so much that was delightful.

We have both experienced a great deal of happiness in our life together so it is possible that my expectations are high.

It would be a great help if you could give me some suggestions as to how to proceed from here. . . .

This letter reveals one or two small problems relating to the writer herself which I would like to clear out of the way before I come to consideration of the husband. First, she is rather overdramatizing the situation. I have never met her or spoken to her, but the fact that she has been through a period of acute depression suggests that she is apt to see certain events in her life in rather sharper and more lurid colors than they are. Her admission that she occasionally falls back on her illness and menopause to provide "a useful excuse when I am not my usual happy self," underlines this. We cannot, any of us, be our usual happy selves *all* the time, but we are not expected to find excuses for our moods. These characteristics have to be taken into account when assessing her complaint against her husband.

Then there is her personal sexual attitude, which seems to me somewhat illogical. The real reason for her writing to me is her sexual frustration arising out of her husband's sexual neglect of her. As she describes this neglect, which is total, there is no wonder that she is feeling sexually frustrated. I, too, am romantic enough to want a sexual relationship illuminated by love, but the physical tensions, which give rise to a very large proportion of the total frustration in *all* cases, can be relieved considerably by masturbation, especially when accompanied by good fantasies. This being so, since she also rejects masturbation, she seems intent on enhancing her martyrdom. She could, therefore, help herself a good deal if she wanted to. On the other hand, her husband has landed her with a sizable problem, and she has every right to complain because the problem need never have arisen.

From her phrase, "Several times over the years my husband has promised to consult his doctor about his impotence, but has never done so," two things emerge: first, the partial impotence from which he is suffering is of some standing—certainly longer than six years, probably eight or nine—and second, that he has done nothing about it, and that whatever may be his reason for this neglect, he has been a sex-lazy husband.

Say he first took refuge in partial impotence nine years ago—this would make him fifty-two. At that age and in his profession he would have been coming under the pressure of the closing phase of his career. He would realize that he had little time left before retirement in which really to make his mark, and I think that if one challenged him with it, he would admit that his reason for dropping out of sex was that his work left him too tired at the end of the day for lovemaking. If one probed deeper one would discover, I am pretty certain, that he had a second line of defense—that he could not be expected to remain as sexually active as he had been when he was younger, because he was beginning to go through "the male climacteric." The male climacteric is nearly always put forward by sex-lazy men in their late fifties and sixties for their lack of sexual activity.

The male climacteric is largely a myth! It is true that as a man gets older his sex drive does become a little less strong, but if he sees to it that he remains sexually active, except that he will not make love quite so frequently, he will have a very adequate and satisfying capacity and performance rating *all* his life.

Those authorities who promote the idea of the male climacteric do men—and women—a serious injustice! As I have said, there is a slowing down of the sex drive as a man gets older which is due to certain changes taking place in his hormone production. The word climacteric is another term for menopause, and knowing this, many men, and particularly sex-lazy men, equate the so-called male climacteric with the female menopause. But, in fact, there is absolutely no comparison. The woman's hormonal changes are extensive; the man's are not. After her menopause the woman can no longer produce her sex-cell (the egg) whereas a man goes on producing sperm-carrying semen all his life, provided he has reasonably good health. Picasso and the master-cellist Pablo Casals both became fathers in their eighties and nineties, a former Bishop of Peterborough when he was seventy-three, and to my personal knowledge several (undistinguished) septuagenarians and octogenarians have performed a similar feat. But even if sperm production ceases, the seminal vesicles and prostate continue to produce their fluids until very late old age, the penis remains capable of erection, and the man capable of orgasm and ejaculation. I had a letter from a gentleman of seventy-eight the other morning who still makes love and finds it intensely satisfying two or three times a week; and I put it in the file with a number of similar letters I have received over the years from men a little younger and some a year or two older.

I am well aware that cases have been recorded of men exhibiting the classic symptoms of the female menopause—hot flushes, depression, irritability, backache, and so on—but I am firmly convinced that the appearance of such symptoms has been psychologically induced. The main thing for the man who realizes that his sex drive is slowing down is not to retreat before it, but to challenge it by engaging in lovemaking as often as he can make the opportunity. The man who accepts the slowing down of his sex drive at fifty-five will be totally sexually inactive by the time he is sixty-five. He will have become impotent and unable to make love because, psychologically, that is what he has chosen to be. It seems that the sex-lazy man knows this instinctively, and he deliberately drops out from sex, because it is the easier line to take.

The wife of the man in his middle fifties who begins to show signs of neglecting making love to her must strike at once as soon as his laziness becomes apparent. She must give him no peace. She must bully him into making love to her. If she does not, then she must not come asking for miracles when the age of miracles is past.

I feel quite sure that something like this has happened to my correspondent and her husband. Maybe he was motivated, too, by an unconscious jealousy of her work outside the home, but fundamentally it was his being allowed to drift into sexual inactivity that caused their present situation. Nor, unfortunately, are they an isolated case. I said earlier, that there are more sex-lazy men in the fifty-five to sixty-five age group than in any other age group. It is one of the things about sex that puzzles me, for when there is a satisfactory sexual relationship in later age, the risk of boredom arising out of retirement is shown to be practically nonexistent. I would have thought, too, that the leisure retirement brings would encourage a greater intimacy between a couple who have spent a lifetime working and bringing up children.

I know I am asking a good deal of women to take their husbands in hand if necessary, because just at the time they should be doing so they will probably be coping with their own menopause. But dare I suggest that such an occupation will, I think, help them to overcome their own difficulties more easily, for many of the woman's menopausal problems spring from the fact that most have too much time to think about themselves.

No woman should tolerate a sex-lazy husband of any variety in any age group. Maybe attempts to correct the situation will lead to difficulties with temper and temperament, but I am sure these need be only temporary. If they do prove permanent then I think one may take it for granted that the relationship is not based on love.

Chapter SEVEN

"My Husband Always Wants to Talk About Sex"

Dear Mr. Chartham: I don't know what to do. My husband is always wanting to talk about sex, and I don't think it's quite nice. I'm twenty-five and he is twenty-eight and we've been married for eighteen months. I was always brought up to think that sex isn't a subject people should talk about. I know that things are changing these days, and that people are much more free in talking about the intimate side of their life, but to me this isn't a change for the good. To be so frank and open seems to me to take away much of the mystery from sex, and without the mystery half the excitement goes out of it. I know that men are very different from women in their outlook on sex, and that among themselves they do talk about it, usually in very crude, coarse terms, but I've never heard of a man talking about it to a woman. Not that my husband uses crude terms, but even when he uses the right words, I feel embarrassed by some of the questions he asks. Surely a man can tell when a woman has her climax, for example? And is there any need for a man to ask a woman when he is making love to her if she is enjoying it, or if he is caressing her in the way she likes to be caressed, or if there is anything she would like him to do which he doesn't do? But it isn't only in bed that he talks. Often he looks across the meal table at me and makes some remark about my breasts. At other times he comes up to me and puts his hands on my buttocks and says, "You've got a great behind honey!" I don't think it's necessary to say things like that, do you? Besides, one of these days we shall have a family, and what if he was to forget himself and say some of these things to me in front of them? I should die of shame. Once or twice I've told him I don't like talking about sex, but each time he just laughed and said, "What a funny, shy, little thing you are!" How can I make him understand that it does embarrass me?

I have to admit that when I first read the opening lines of this letter I was a bit taken aback, because I did not appreciate that there are people about these days of this young woman's age who have been brought up to the view that sex is not a subject one should talk about and, moreover, young people of her generation who believe that there should be mystery surrounding sex. But I ought not to have been surprised, because many letters to me begin, "Dear Mr. Chartham, I hope you will be able to understand what I am going to try to say in this letter, because I don't know the right words to use . . ." or, "Dear Mr. Chartham, I hope I shan't embarrass you, or you will think me coarse, but if I don't express myself in the only way I know how, I might just as well not try to write to you at all, and I hope you will understand how difficult it is when you haven't been taught how to put things."

I also should not have been surprised, really, because I am daily having it driven home to me that far too many married couples are still going through the whole of their married lives without saying a single word to one another on the subject of sex. I am well aware, too, that many couples who run into sexual difficulties would not have done so if only they had talked to one another about what was bothering them sexually.

In fact, one of my oft-repeated cries is *Communicate! Communicate! Communicate!*

Of course there are some difficulties about talking to one another about sex which arise solely from the lack of a socially acceptable word. The Latin words—*vagina, clitoris, penis, scrotum, testicles,* and so on—have an artificiality about them which puts people who know them off using them, while *sexual intercourse, the sex act, coitus, orgasm,* and *intromission* are so pompous and stilted that people say they would feel foolish using them. The four-letter words, which were once perfectly respectable and are good, strong, no-nonsense words of Anglo-Saxon origin, are still taboo, though there are signs that they are recovering their respectability. (I hope, personally, that the time is near when they will become everyday words again.) Nevertheless, there are many men who, out of what I think is a mistaken sense of propriety, cannot bring themselves to use them even to their wives, while there are many women who, if they knew the words, wouldn't dream of using them lest they undermine their reputation for decency or affront their feminine modesty.

Yet it cannot be stressed too strongly that men and women must learn to talk to one another frankly and fully about their sexual activities and experiences. So what to do about the language problem?

You will have probably noticed by reading the book so far, and if you have read any of my other books, that with one or two exceptions, I have been able to devise words and phrases that are not unacceptable; e.g., *to come*, to reach orgasm; *lovemaking,* for sexual intercourse; *coupling,* for intromission, i.e., insertion of the penis in the vagina; *vaginal lips,* for labia, vulva. These terms, I like to think, are everyday and down to earth, but are quite suitable for use between men and women. But I am still stuck with penis, scrotum, testicles, vagina, and clitoris. I cannot for the life of me think why husbands and wives should not use the four-letter equivalents for *penis, testicles,* and *vagina* in their private conversations, but I do realize that it may take a little getting used to, though I am sure that any embarrassment will be only temporary. However, there is another way, though some may find the idea rather whimsical.

Two young friends of mine, former history students, who have now trained themselves to use the four-letter words quite naturally between themselves and like-minded friends, in the first two or three years of their relationship referred to the *penis* as William, the *vagina* as Mary, the *clitoris* as Prince William, and the *testicles* as gemini (twins). They avoided the use of scrotum altogether, because, they said, "according to the phrasing you use, gemini can stand for scrotum as well as testicles." This is an idea which I throw out. The terms or words used need not have historical connections; couples can invent their own personal phrases.

Now let me quote my reply to my correspondent.

Dear Mrs.———: Thank you for your letter. You don't know how lucky you are to have a husband who wants to talk to you about sex. If talking about sex is not nice, then sex itself cannot be nice; and I feel quite certain that you do not agree with that.

One of the great mistakes our Victorian ancestors made was to surround sex with a veil of mystery. No one talked to anyone about it; young people were left to find out about it as best they could, and almost without exception they learned of it in the worst possible way—in the gutter terms to which sex had been relegated. They also acquired a lot of wrong information. Women, as a rule, did not learn much at all. Large numbers of young women entered marriage without any idea of how men and women couple, and because their husbands had not learned anything about loveplay in their gutter-school, most of these women bore large families of children and went through the whole of their married lives without knowing what a climax was, or even that they were capable of having one. The consequence of all this mystery, as I say, was to make sex a dirty thing, and certainly something that no "nice" women should enjoy, when it should be something beautiful, satisfying and full of fun and laughter, as it must be if we use physical lovemaking as the expression of the love we have for our partner. I just can't understand what you mean when you say "without the mystery half the excitement goes out of sex."

The crux of the matter is that to make sex exciting and as pleasurable and satisfying as possible, there must be *no* mystery. Not only must there be no mystery, there must be a great deal of knowledge about one's partner's body and about one's own. We must know what makes us tick sexually, and what makes our partner tick sexually. We must know this so that we can provide ourselves and our partner with the highest degree of pleasure, both physically and mentally, as a result of our lovemaking. Lovemaking is not only a partnership, it is an *equal* partnership. This is a widely accepted view these days. The times are past when the woman could lie back and let her partner make love to her, without lifting a finger to make love to him in return. He cannot enjoy lovemaking as much as he should unless he is fondled, caressed, and aroused as much as he caresses, fondles, and arouses his partner.

Now, it is quite impossible for either a man or a woman to know by instinct what sexually pleases the

"MY HUSBAND ALWAYS WANTS TO TALK ABOUT SEX" 87

partner most. I know that there are books available to guide a couple in this respect—I have written a number of them myself—but a book can only give general lines of guidance. We all differ so much from one another in our responses to sexual stimulation that one cannot really say that any two people are sexually alike. To give just a simple example: I get very excited if my nipples are caressed by my partner, but a good friend of mine finds caressing of his nipples off-putting, it merely tickles him.

How then do a couple find out how the partner can be most stimulated? By experiment? That may take years. On the other hand, a word or two need only take a minute or two. I know a woman whose husband used to suck the lobes of her ears while making love to her, because he had read in a book that women find it stimulating. Many women do, but she was one of those who were left absolutely cold by it. Instead of telling him he was wasting his time—good time which he could have spent on more effective caresses—she suffered it in silence for a couple of years more, getting more and more irritated each time, until she eventually lost her temper, snapped at him, gave him the fright of his life, and involved them in the first serious quarrel they had had.

Your husband has got the right idea. He is, I think, trying to find out what you enjoy most, and instead of wishing he wouldn't, you should encourage him to ask even more questions, and you should ask him as many. (By the way, some women, though completely satisfied by their climax, do not react in such a way that the man can tell when they have come. When your husband asks you if you have come, he is showing concern that you have been satisfied. He might not bother to make sure, and you might never come at all.) Mind you, as the years go by, and you gain more and more knowledge about your partner's body, you will not have to ask him so many questions, nor he ask you so many, because regular lovemaking will have shown you what most pleases him and you. But lovemaking must never, at any time of life, after thirty years as well as after one, cease to be a continuous experiment. There is plenty of scope, if you have the imagination, and only by this means can you avoid falling foul of the greatest enemy of sexual happiness—boredom. Nothing encourages boredom so easily or quickly as a routine of lovemaking followed every time. It does not matter that you are sexually satisfied by your routine, soon you will find that mere physical satisfaction is not enough, and as soon as you make the discovery, even the satisfaction you do get will pall. Not only that, every year that goes by sees changes taking place in our bodies. These changes alter our responses so there is a constant need throughout life to experiment, and experimenting means talking.

I really do not understand your objections to his admiring remarks about your figure. Mostly I get complaints from wives that their husbands don't seem to notice them. You should be delighted that he not only notices your figure, but that it excites him. It is the best insurance you have against his looking elsewhere for excitement. The husband who flatters is the husband who knows on which side his bread is buttered.

As for your fear that he may do or say things in front of the children—I'm all for it. It does children no end of good to know without a doubt that their parents love one another. It gives them a sense of security that nothing else can. As they grow older, it does them just as much good to realize that Mom and Dad are sexually happy. Love and sex then tie up, and this is what it is really all about.

I know it may be difficult for you at first to overcome your embarrassment about talking about sex, but do believe me, he is on the right lines. Stop sheltering behind your feminine false modesty, because unless you do you will sooner or later regret it. Once you have taken the plunge, you will find that your embarrassment will soon wear off, especially as you have such an easy husband to talk to. You will also find that sex without any mystery is much more exciting than sex with mystery.

Best wishes.

Nor is it a matter of talking about sex in order to become a more expert lover. Lovemaking should not be a dance without music. It can be, of course, but silent lovemaking, which is nearly always performed in darkness as well, always strikes me as being a kind of invisible puppet show, with the partners going through the motions. Puppets don't cease to be puppets when their manipulators speak for them. Voiceless, they remain inanimate objects. A couple making love should be alive, with a quality of aliveness that they display in no other activity.

Talking during lovemaking should not be confined to putting the partner right about how he is doing, it should also include appreciation for the sensations he is producing in you and that you are producing in him. I think there must be very few indeed who do express their appreciation during lovemaking, who do not find it extremely stimulating. There is no need to go into long and flowing compliments, nor to keep up a constant flow, but a fairly often repeated, "Yes, yes!" or "That's good," or "Go on doing that," or "You're wonderful" is quite sufficient to add many degrees of physical pleasure through the mental stimulus they provide.

There is one word of warning I think I should give. Very many men as their sensations increase, and especially after they have coupled and are about to come, for reasons too involved to need explanation here, exclaim, "No, no, oh, no!" Actually they mean, "Oh yes! Yes, please!" So do not be put off if your partner gives these cries and don't stop doing what you are doing because you imagine you must be hurting him. Incidentally, if he tries to get away from your hands, don't let him, unless at the same time he quietly and calmly asks you to stop for a moment or two. This trying to escape you is the same kind of reaction which makes him exclaim "No," when he really means "Yes." If you let him get away, he will be very disappointed because it is the mock-resistance he is making that is arousing him even more. On the other hand, if he draws away and quietly asks you to stop whatever it is you are doing, stop at once! It means that you have brought him on too far, and if you continue you will make him come prematurely.

Some women talk automatically while being made love to, and a number of them use the most extraordinary language. Not long ago I received a letter from a disturbed young bridegroom, who, after one night of love, was wondering whether he might not have made a mistake in marrying his wife. They were engaged four months before they married, and during that time they did not make love. He was twenty-three and she was twenty. She had been quite honest with him, and told him that she was not a virgin. They were lent a cottage in the depths of the country for their honeymoon, which meant several hours of driving after the reception. They were so tired when they reached the cottage that they decided to go to bed at once, and they were so exhausted that they did not even attempt to make love, which was very wise of them. They did not wake up until late, to find it raining hard and being generally miserable outside. She got a tray of coffee and toast and they breakfasted in bed. When they had finished they made love for the first time.

I found when I began to make love to her [he wrote] that she was already excited. As soon as I touched her she began to gasp for breath and moan. I was so excited that when she touched me after a minute or two, I came. This seemed to upset her quite a bit, and she kept caressing me, trying to keep my erection going, and sort of half-whispering, half-moaning, "Please come back, darling, please come back. Please love me." And things like that.

Well, I got another erection quite quickly and went on making love to her, but in a very short time she asked me to go into her, and practically pulled me on top of her. As I began to move, she threw back her head with her eyes closed, and began to breathe very heavily until her breath was coming in a kind of shrill hissing, and saliva kept bubbling over her lips. I asked her if she was all right, and she said, rather angrily I thought, "Of course I am." After another minute or two she began to jerk and put her hands on my shoulders, and tried to push me away, but when I did begin to move away, because I thought I might be hurting her, she crossed her legs over the small of my back so that I couldn't move off her, but still kept pushing my shoulders away, saying loudly, "Fight me, you bastard! Fight me!"

Well, I took her at her word, and the more she pushed me away, the more I pushed into her, and let my whole weight go on to her. All the time she kept squirming and wriggling as though she was trying to get away, and cursing, using the most filthy language. I'm not a prude really, but I don't much care to hear women using four-letter words.

I don't know how long it was before she came, but when she did, she let out a scream, went entirely rigid for a second or two, then collapsed and lay quite still. I came a moment or two later, and as I lay panting on top of her, because it had been really quite a fight, she opened her eyes, smiled, and kissed me and stroked my hair and said, "That was glorious, darling. Was it good for you, too?"

I said yes, and so it had been, but my mind was just in a wild confusion. She is a gentle girl to all outward appearances, gay, kind, generous, and with a wonderful sense of humor. She comes from a very nice home, and her parents are kind, pleasant, quiet people. What upset me more than her wanting me more or less to rape her, was the words she used. If you had asked me, I would have sworn that she did not know half of them. Some of the things she said would have been quite high for a football locker room.

You said in *Husband & Lover* that some highly sexed women squirm and moan and often shout, but you didn't say that they used really filthy language. That's what's really upsetting me. Is she really a licentious girl, with a rather dirty mind? Mind you, except when she gets terribly excited when we're making love—and it doesn't *always* happen, though it happens quite frequently—she's her usual sweet, gentle self, and never utters a hint of dirt. But is she play-acting when she's like this, and only her real self comes out when she loses control of herself sexually? What I'm afraid of is that if she's her real self during lovemaking, she may not bother to go on play-acting. I know you said that highly sexed women could react with groans and cries, and even back-scratching, and I don't mean to be critical, but you didn't give any idea of what some can really be like. You see, besides the language and the violence, she's not too easy to satisfy. I can keep going while she comes two or three times, but I don't know how long I can go on keeping going when she wants it almost—though not quite—every day.

Is there anything that can be done to quieten her down a bit, and what do you think her chances are of developing into a foul-mouthed woman, who will someday say something awful in front of our minister? Mind you, when she's normal, she's as adorable as ever, is kind and gentle and considerate, and everything I always imagined a wife should be . . . . Don't be long in letting me know what you think, please! Have I made a ghastly mistake?

No, he had not made a ghastly mistake, I was able to tell him. Some women have been reacting this way to lovemaking probably since men and women arrived on the planet. Seigneur Pierre de Brantome, the sixteenth-century soldier and writer of scandalous memoirs, who in 1561 accompanied Mary Queen of Scots from France to Holyrood, wrote what has now become a famous erotic classic, *The Lives of Gallant Ladies*. In a chapter entitled *Of Lovers' Speech* he has gone into this phenomenon known by psychiatrists as *erotolalia*. "I have heard it said [he wrote] by many great knights and gallant gentlemen who have lain with great ladies that they have found them a hundred times more dissolute and lewd in speech than common women and such."

As the young man said about his wife, one wonders how such nice, quiet, gentle, well-bred women have learned the four-letter words and other colorful language they use. Some of them are unaware that they do use such language, and those who are aware are unable to explain anything, except that they cannot resist letting rip as they do, however much they try not to. If you are one of these women, neither you nor your partner need be afraid that you will address your minister in the same language. This has never been known to happen.

Nor is erotolalia confined to women. Men can react in the same way, though where they learned the language they use is not so much of a mystery. So, if your partner assaults your ears with words you scarcely know exist, or have only a vague inkling of, don't blame him, don't imagine he is gratuitously insulting you. He can't help it. In his unexcited moments he will be ashamed of himself and deeply apologetic. Tell him not to worry, and accept his apologies gracefully.

Don't confine your words of appreciation to his techniques: admire his body, too. Tell him you have never seen such muscled thighs, such rippling muscles in a belly, such a big and beautiful penis, nor such a strong erection. He will respond with pride, because you have admired his manhood, and made him feel really good by flattering his sexual ego, and he will reciprocate in kind. You will have the most glorious breasts in creation, the softest skin, the most agile thighs, the most welcoming of all vaginas: and you will feel good, too.

But while, in my view, it is essential that a couple should talk while having sex and about sex, it is most essential when they run into sexual difficulties. This can happen occasionally even in the happiest relationships. It is surprising, however, even when a couple have been used to talking about their lovemaking, how they are somehow inhibited from discussing their own or the partner's little problems. As a consequence, the longer they hesitate to bring what is worrying them out into the open, the more difficult they make the ultimate solution.

Nearly all sexual difficulties can be dispelled by the cooperation of a pertinent and understanding partner. But no partner can cooperate if the one with the difficulty will not talk about it. And when they do talk, it must be as fully and as frankly as possible. The couple who do not customarily talk about sex must make a real effort to do so if they do run up against a problem, and this applies especially to the late middle-aged because they can more easily drop out of sex than younger couples, and blight what should be the happy evening of their lives.

May I beg you, then, never to refuse to talk to your husband about any aspect of sex? May I beg you, equally earnestly, to make him talk to you if he shows no signs of doing so himself? Get into the habit of doing this from the first moment that your relationship looks like becoming a permanent one; don't put it off until you are married; because the younger you are the easier it is.

If you are already clocking up several years of married life and have not yet begun to talk, please don't hesitate a moment longer. Please believe me, it is merely a matter of overcoming initial embarrassment, of taking the plunge. Once you have jumped in, you will be wondering whatever was it that held you back.

Remember the slogan for all couples with regard to sex: *Communicate, communicate, communicate!*

Chapter EIGHT

Being the Active Partner

For the last twenty years at least, this has been one of my favorite hobbyhorses. In all my books, and in a good many articles, I have drummed home, drummed away at what I believe to be the right concept of the marriage (and, therefore, the sexual) relationship, i.e., that it is not only a partnership, but an *equal* partnership.

An *equal* partnership carries *equal* responsibilities. When it comes to lovemaking, then, the woman has the responsibility to see that the man enjoys the experience and obtains the most satisfaction that it is possible for him to obtain after making allowances for the mood he is in, and other circumstances of the lovemaking. In order to fulfil this responsibility, the woman can no longer be the passive partner, lying there, submitting her body to her partner's caresses, and making no return for it. Her hands must wander, fondle and caress, her lips and her tongue must go exploring; and what hands, lips and tongue encounter they must know how to inflame with sensations.

When Dr. Marie Stopes rediscovered the orgasm for women half a century ago she did not realize, I think, the extent to which she was exposing women to sex. Marie Stopes had a very unhappy and sexually unsatisfactory first marriage, and though her second one to A. V. Roe, the aircraft designer, turned out to be just the opposite, she never really forgave her first husband, and reflected this continuing bitterness in the role in lovemaking that she allocated to men.

She lost a great opportunity to emancipate women sexually and fully way back there in the 1920's, when she did not reveal to women that they are sexually equal with men. Using the traditional male role of hunter and aggressor in sex to obtain for women their experience of the orgasm, at the same time she sought to avenge herself for all the sexual unhappiness she had suffered at the hands of one man, and she succeeded. By placing the whole responsibility for the woman achieving orgasm on the man, she has produced more unhappiness among husbands, wives, and lovers than anyone else who has worked in the field of sex education. "*He* must bring you to orgasm!" she told women, "and if he doesn't, it proves what an incompetent lover he is!" This dictum has generated more feelings of sexual inadequacy among men, and consequently more sexual misery among couples, than any other. Marie Stopes intended to punish men, and her bitterness against them blinded her to the inevitable result, that if she made men feel inferior, they would not be able to produce the pleasure and satisfaction she taught women to demand, and so increased suffering all round. By concentrating on the orgasm and overlooking the tremendous experience that mutual loveplay properly performed can be, she postponed women's sexual liberation for half a century. Let me try to explain how.

The Victorians had regarded women as sexless creatures in the sense that they were denied sexual feelings. No nice women would ever admit that making love was pleasant and rewarding. (For the majority, it never was.) Men, made as they were, needed sex, and though women did not, they nevertheless had to submit to the experience for the relief of men's sexual needs. But though they had to submit, they did not have to know anything about practical sex. In fact, any woman who knew the first thing about practical sex could not be a nice woman. When sex, for the majority of couples, consisted only of penis-vagina contact and the male orgasm and ejaculation, there was not much to know, but even the rudimentary knowledge of how penis-vagina contact was achieved was the sole concern of men. "Don't worry about that!" mothers told their daughters. "He will know what to do. Sex is for men, not for nice women!" This was what Marie Stopes failed to eliminate from women's minds, and though admittedly she did advocate that sex should be pleasurable and enjoyable, she placed the entire burden for seeing that it is on men. Consequently, we still have today many hundreds of thousands of women coming to marriage still ignorant of what sex is all about, except that they will be required to lie on their backs and their husband will put his penis into them.

This pathetic letter arrived on my desk the other morning.

Dear Dr. Chartham: Will you please help me? I am nearly forty-five years old and my husband is forty-eight. We have been married twenty-seven years and have seven children whose ages range from nine months to twenty-five years. Until six months ago I knew nothing about orgasm. I've never had a climax with my husband.

I saw a magazine in a friend's house. It contained an article on orgasm. Also it mentioned masturbation, which I didn't know was possible for women, and the clitoris, which I didn't even know I had. I tried masturbating, and after several days I had orgasm. I told my husband and he has tried to help me, but with no success. I have always enjoyed lovemaking, though I've always asked my husband to make it last longer and been a little disappointed when he finished. Now I know what should happen, it has spoiled things for both of us. I want to talk to my doctor, but cannot bring myself to do so. He is a very religious man and wouldn't even let me have an abortion last year, although I was very upset when I became pregnant. I cannot take the Pill as it makes me bleed badly and gives me bad pains in my back and stomach, so I am to be fitted with the coil. Will this affect my chances of orgasm during intercourse? Am I likely to have this pleasure at all now? I feel terribly cheated. Two friends I have spoken to have also never had an orgasm and didn't know any more about it than I did.

I have read that you help couples who have difficulties. Even if I knew where to go I would not have courage to go in a sex-shop. My husband has agreed that I should write to you. I hope you will write to us soon.

It seems incredible that in this day and age there are women—and men, for that matter—who do not know that women have a clitoris, let alone what it is for. Obviously, too, there are people about who have never heard of Marie Stopes, which is a good thing, because that makes my task easier. But it is, nevertheless, extremely sad that a woman can be so ignorant of her sexual function that she has deprived herself of pleasure all these years. It also shows that it is not much good "leaving sex" to some men. They may know the rudiments, but in sex the rudiments are just not enough. As I see it, there is no stronger argument for women making themselves knowledgeable about sex, if only to protect them against ignorant men.

But actually there is a much greater necessity for women to make themselves knowledgeable about sex. If lovemaking is to be an *equal* partnership the whole former concept of it changes.

Loveplay, his skills in the techniques of which determines a man's status as a lover, has been devised to close the arousal-gap, i.e., the difference in speed of the man's and the woman's response to stimulation. The skillful male lover knows that according to the various caresses he applies to his partner the more intensely will she come and the greater pleasure and satisfaction she will ultimately have. Women who have not been told so, and a very large number of men themselves, are not aware that if men are made love to in a way similar to the way in which they make love to women, i.e., by caressing and fondling their sensitive zones and other techniques, the man's orgasm sensations, his pleasure and satisfaction can also be very greatly intensified.

Now, if lovemaking is used to express the emotional love that the partners have for one another—and I repeat that in my view this is the most satisfactory reason for making love—then the object of lovemaking must be to induce the most pleasant experience and most intense orgasm sensations that skills make possible, because only in this way can the true depth of emotional love be expressed. This requires that the woman shall take just as active a part in lovemaking as the man, because if she does not she cannot be expressing the depth of her love for her partner. She must, therefore, become as skilled a lover as he is, and if she fails to provide him with a memorable experience, she must also accept the slur of being a failure as a lover, just as Marie Stopes advised her to condemn her partner if he did not bring her to orgasm every time they made love.

In order to be a skillful lover, she must learn his sensitive zones, and the types of caresses and the particular parts of his body that provide him with the greatest sensual thrills. This means experimenting and exploring, which in turn means that she must regard his body as her own. Not only that, if she is going to express her love in its true depth, she must do her very best to overcome any inhibitions she may have, and particularly with regard to oral intercourse, which, I think I can say without exaggerating, all men not only enjoy, but deeply appreciate and have specially warm feelings for the partner who will engage in it without fuss.

All right then—sex is not only for women, it is also for *nice* women, women who love their husbands and want to express their love in a way that can leave no doubt in the partner's mind. Every session of lovemaking should be designed to this end. On the other hand, this does not mean that the woman has to be as active as the man at every session of lovemaking. There are occasions when she should lie back and let her partner make love to her, without her doing much in return. If the partner is in a specially passionate mood—and the experienced woman can always tell this—he will want to show her how much he loves her by excelling himself in his techniques of arousal. If she wants to join in, in any case, it may be fatal, because when a man is under the influence of a really *grand passion*, it takes very little to make him come, and a half a dozen caresses may be sufficient to spoil everything. So let him do all the "work" on occasion, for not only will you be showing your love for him by letting him take you over completely, you will also be getting variation into your love, which is essential if you are to keep boredom at bay.

But marriage is an *equal* partnership, and if you from time to time let him make love to you as I have just described, he must also let you make love to him in the same fashion. He must lie passively, while you play the active role from the beginning of loveplay right through to climax. He may perhaps fondle your nipples or caress your clitoris, if he can reach it; but he must let you do whatever you want without lifting a finger to help you, unless you specifically ask him to.

I have always advocated, ever since I began to press the concept of marriage as an *equal* partnership, that if a woman is sexually roused and wants to make love, but her partner shows no sign of doing so, she is absolutely justified in starting lovemaking and remaining the active partner throughout. Equally, he must cooperate by letting her do so. There are very few men indeed who cannot be roused and thoroughly enjoy the whole experience, even when the nearest thought of sex was a million miles away. The really weary man can respond if his partner knows what she is about, and as I explained in a previous chapter, can experience total relaxation as a result.

Now I am going a step further and advocating that the

paperback booksmith

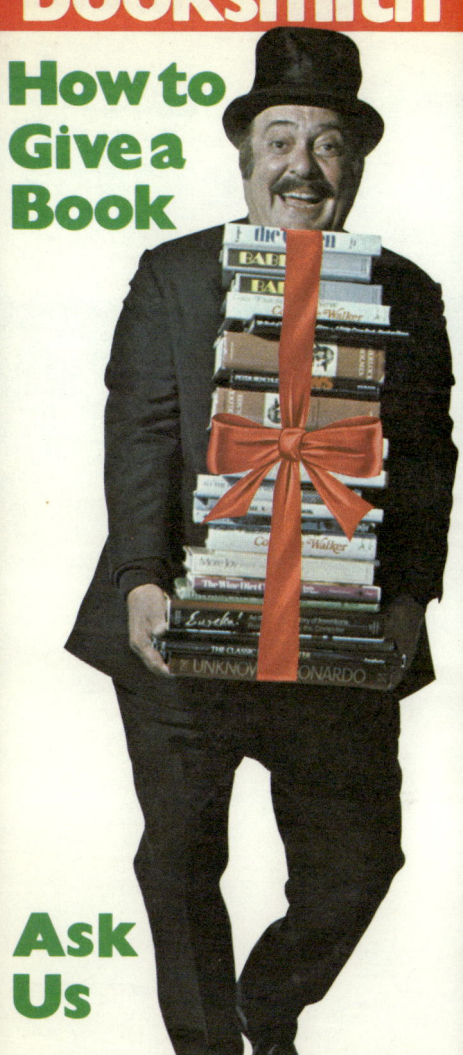

How to Give a Book

Ask Us

OXFORD VALLEY MALL
Langhorne, Pa. (215) 752-1555
And Stores Throughout the Eastern United States

paperback booksmith

"Dedicated to the fine art of browsing"

Massachusetts

Boston
(617) 536-4433
(617) 267-7515
Brookline ★
(617) 566-6660
Cambridge ★
(617) 864-2321
Chelmsford ★
(617) 256-3514
Chestnut Hill ★
(617) 244-6036
Chicopee ★
Danvers
(617) 777-1064
Dedham ★
(617) 329-2880
Fall River ★
(617) 678-6388
Hadley ★
(413) 584-2045
Hanover ★
(617) 826-4520
Hyannis ★
(617) 775-6566
Natick
(617) 655-3033
Springfield ★
(413) 543-4434
Worcester ★
(617) 752-9068

Florida

Boca Raton
(305) 368-1300
Jacksonville
(904) 388-4091
Lakeland
(813) 688-9444
North Palm Beach ★
(305) 844-7770
St. Petersburg ★
(813) 522-7486
Seminole ★
(813) 393-5900
South Daytona ★
(904) 761-3792

New Jersey

Plainfield
(201) 753-4415
Vineland ★
(609) 327-2605
Wayne
(201) 785-0751

New York

Baldwinsville ★
(315) 638-2666
Colonie ★
(518) 459-9336
Massapequa ★
(516) 795-3090
Mohegan Lake
(914) 528-1229
Staten Island
(212) 761-4414
Yonkers
(914) 969-3440

Pennsylvania

Bradford ★
(814) 362-4974
Camp Hill I ★
Cornwells Heights
(215) 638-7780
Langhorne
(215) 752-1555
Scranton
(717) 346-9162
Wilkes-Barre ★
(717) 824-7373

Connecticut

Ansonia ★
(203) 734-0789
New London ★
(203) 442-1780
Simsbury ★
(203) 658-9664

New Hampshire

Bedford ★
(603) 669-7583
Nashua ★
(603) 889-9202
Portsmouth ★
(603) 431-5120

Maryland

Baltimore
(301) 285-7914
Lanham ★
(301) 459-0009

Indiana

Richmond ★

★ **Records Too!**

paperback booksmith

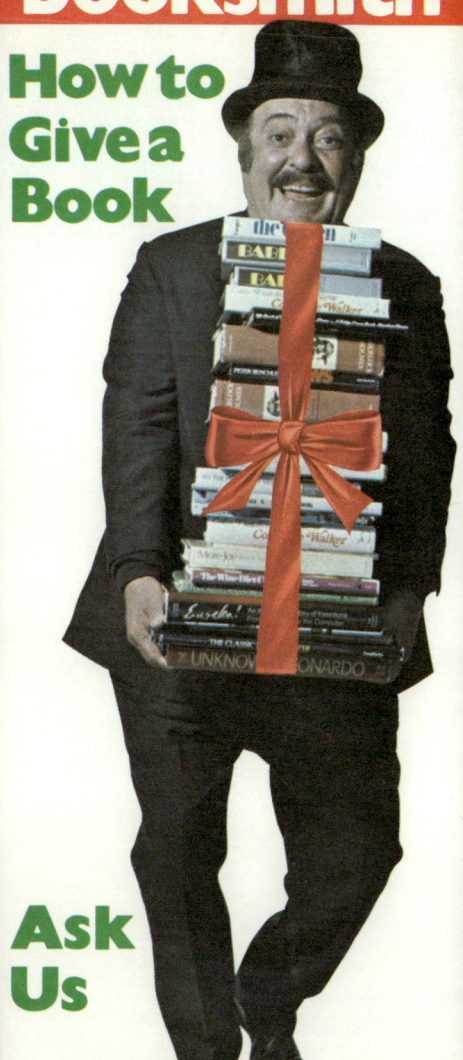

How to Give a Book

Ask Us

OXFORD VALLEY MALL
Langhorne, Pa. (215) 752-1555
And Stores Throughout the Eastern United States

paperback booksmith

"Dedicated to the fine art of browsing"

Massachusetts

Boston
(617) 536-4433
(617) 267-7515
Brookline★
(617) 566-6660
Cambridge★
(617) 864-2321
Chelmsford★
(617) 256-3514
Chestnut Hill★
(617) 244-6036
Chicopee★
Danvers
(617) 777-1064
Dedham★
(617) 329-2880
Fall River★
(617) 678-6388
Hadley★
(413) 584-2045
Hanover★
(617) 826-4520
Hyannis★
(617) 775-6566
Natick
(617) 655-3033
Springfield★
(413) 543-4434
Worcester★
(617) 752-9068

Florida

Boca Raton
(305) 368-1300
Jacksonville
(904) 388-4091
Lakeland
(813) 688-9444
North Palm Beach★
(305) 844-7770
St. Petersburg★
(813) 522-7486
Seminole★
(813) 393-5900
South Daytona★
(904) 761-3792

New Jersey

Plainfield
(201) 753-4415
Vineland★
(609) 327-2605
Wayne
(201) 785-0751

New York

Baldwinsville★
(315) 638-2666
Colonie★
(518) 459-9336
Massapequa★
(516) 795-3090
Mohegan Lake
(914) 528-1229
Staten Island
(212) 761-4414
Yonkers
(914) 969-3440

Pennsylvania

Bradford★
(814) 362-4974
Camp Hilll★
Cornwells Heights
(215) 638-7780
Langhorne
(215) 752-1555
Scranton
(717) 346-9162
Wilkes-Barre★
(717) 824-7373

Connecticut

Ansonia★
(203) 734-0789
New London★
(203) 442-1780
Simsbury★
(203) 658-9664

New Hampshire

Bedford★
(603) 669-7583
Nashua★
(603) 889-9202
Portsmouth★
(603) 431-5120

Maryland

Baltimore
(301) 285-7914
Lanham★
(301) 459-0009

Indiana

Richmond★

★ **Records Too!**

paperback booksmith

How to Give a Book

Ask Us

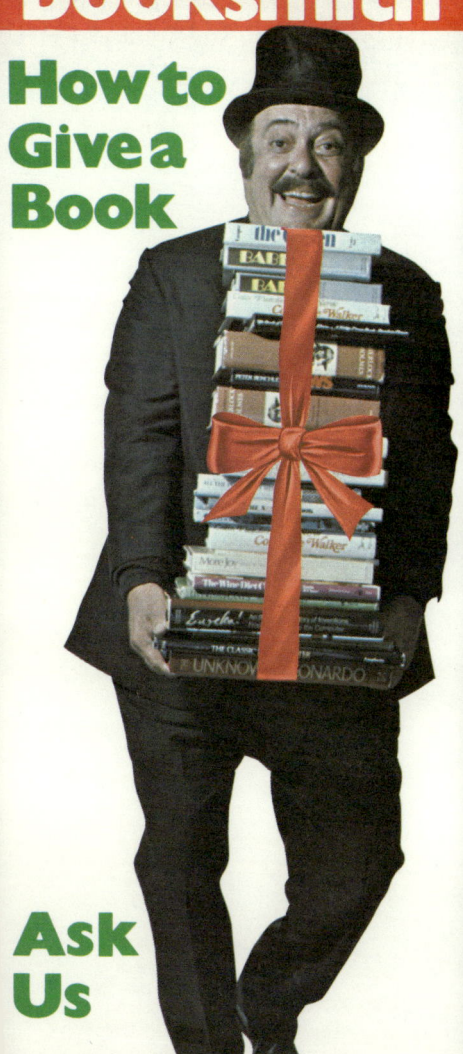

OXFORD VALLEY MALL
Langhorne, Pa. (215) 752-1555
And Stores Throughout the Eastern United States

paperback booksmith

"Dedicated to the fine art of browsing"

Massachusetts

Boston
(617) 536-4433
(617) 267-7515
Brookline *
(617) 566-6660
Cambridge *
(617) 864-2321
Chelmsford *
(617) 256-3514
Chestnut Hill *
(617) 244-6036
Chicopee *
Danvers
(617) 777-1064
Dedham *
(617) 329-2880
Fall River *
(617) 678-6388
Hadley *
(413) 584-2045
Hanover *
(617) 826-4520
Hyannis *
(617) 775-6566
Natick
(617) 655-3033
Springfield *
(413) 543-4434
Worcester *
(617) 752-9068

Florida

Boca Raton
(305) 368-1300
Jacksonville
(904) 388-4091
Lakeland
(813) 688-9444
North Palm Beach *
(305) 844-7770
St. Petersburg *
(813) 522-7486
Seminole *
(813) 393-5900
South Daytona *
(904) 761-3792

New Jersey

Plainfield
(201) 753-4415
Vineland *
(609) 327-2605
Wayne
(201) 785-0751

New York

Baldwinsville *
(315) 638-2666
Colonie *
(518) 459-9336
Massapequa *
(516) 795-3090
Mohegan Lake
(914) 528-1229
Staten Island
(212) 761-4414
Yonkers
(914) 969-3440

Pennsylvania

Bradford *
(814) 362-4974
Camp Hilll *
Cornwells Heights
(215) 638-7780
Langhorne
(215) 752-1555
Scranton
(717) 346-9162
Wilkes-Barre *
(717) 824-7373

Connecticut

Ansonia *
(203) 734-0789
New London *
(203) 442-1780
Simsbury *
(203) 658-9664

New Hampshire

Bedford *
(603) 669-7583
Nashua *
(603) 889-9202
Portsmouth *
(603) 431-5120

Maryland

Baltimore
(301) 285-7914
Lanham *
(301) 459-0009

Indiana

Richmond *

* Records Too!

paperback booksmith

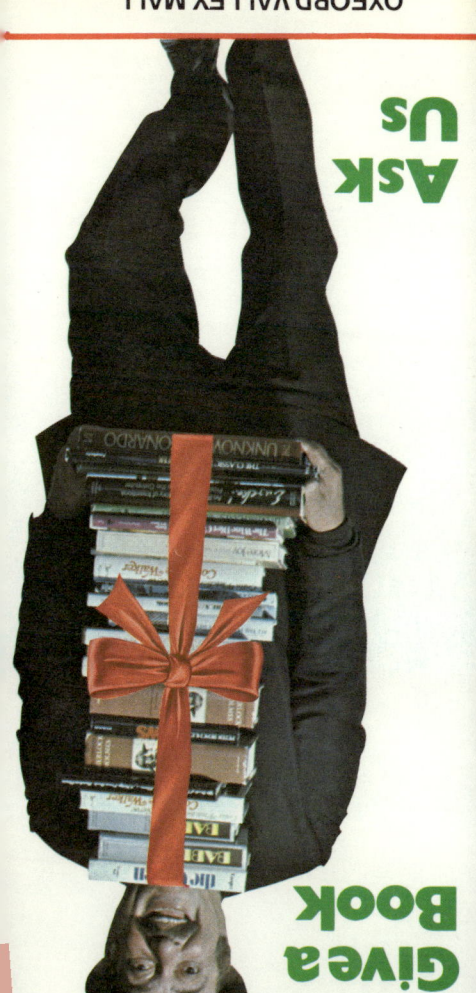

How to Give a Book

Ask Us

OXFORD VALLEY MALL
Langhorne, Pa. (215) 752-1555
And Stores Throughout the Eastern United States

paperback bookmsith

"Dedicated to the fine art of browsing"

Massachusetts

Boston
(617) 536-4433
Brookline
(617) 267-7515
Cambridge
(617) 566-6660
Chestnut Hill *
(617) 864-2321
Chelmsford
(617) 256-3514
Chicopee *
(617) 244-6036
Danvers
(617) 777-1064
Dedham *
(617) 329-2880
Fall River
(617) 678-6388
Hadley *
(413) 584-2045
Hanover *
(617) 826-4520
Hyannis
(617) 775-6566
Natick
(617) 655-3033
Springfield *
(413) 543-4434
Worcester
(617) 752-9068

Florida

Boca Raton
(305) 368-1300
Jacksonville
(904) 388-4091
Lakeland
(813) 688-9444
North Palm Beach *
(305) 844-7770
St. Petersburg
(813) 522-7486
Seminole
(813) 393-5900
South Daytona *
(904) 761-3792

New Jersey

Plainfield
(201) 753-4415

Indiana

Richmond *

Records Too!

New York

Baldwinsville *
(315) 638-2666
Colonie *
(518) 459-9336
Massapequa *
(516) 795-3090
Mohegan Lake
(914) 528-1229
Staten Island
(212) 761-4414
Yonkers
(914) 966-3440

Pennsylvania

Bradford *
(814) 362-4974
Camp Hill *
Cornwells Heights
(215) 638-7780
Langhorne
(215) 752-1555
Scranton
(717) 346-9162
Wilkes-Barre
(717) 824-7373

Connecticut

Ansonia *
(203) 734-0789
New London *
(203) 442-1780
Simsbury *
(203) 658-9664

New Hampshire

Bedford *
(603) 669-7583
Nashua *
(603) 889-9202
Portsmouth *
(603) 431-5120

Maryland

Baltimore
(301) 285-7914
Lanham *
(301) 459-0009

Wayne
(201) 785-0751

woman need not wait for such occasions as these, but is entitled to take over the active role any time she feels like it. Even if her partner has already initiated lovemaking, and the whim takes her, all she has to say is, "Lie still, darling, and let *me* love *you*." I am making this suggestion, because in the past eighteen months countless women have told me that they have this urge from time to time, and ask me if there is anything wrong in them having this desire.

If you have a sexually sophisticated partner he will raise no objections, not only because he recognizes and accepts your right to it, but because most, if not all, men find it both pleasant and exciting to be made love to now and again. On the other hand, you may have a partner like the woman who wrote to me the following letter:

> Dear Dr. Chartham: In *Mainly For Wives* you said that if a woman wants to make love and her husband shows no signs of wanting to, she has every right to be the active partner from beginning to end. There are frequent occasions when I feel I would like to do this with my husband, but he just won't cooperate. He says it's the man's job to make love, not the woman's, and that if he doesn't want to make love that's that. He's even suggested that I'm a bit kinky for even getting the idea. But I can't be, can I, because you say it's all right? What can I do to get him to change his mind?

There is a problem here, because unless a man with such views, mistaken though they are, can be gently persuaded to change them, he can be, so to speak, thrown out of gear. What can happen is that he may find his passivity so out of line with his traditional idea of the male role in sex—the hunter, the leader, the lover—that if he is compelled to accept it against his will he may feel that he is being sexually inadequate. As I explained in a previous chapter, feelings of inadequacy can play such havoc with his performance that he may become unable to get an erection, or if he does, it may fade at just the crucial moment.

So what can be done? I think that the only safe way to attempt it is to stress that you want to show him how very much you love him. Flatter him by telling him that he is an absolutely wonderful lover, none better. At the same time, though, you don't see why he should always have to do all the work. It isn't that you want to usurp his role, it's just that you want to demonstrate your love for him more fully than he lets you have a chance of showing it when he is making love with you.

Somehow you will have to strike a balance between appearing to be too eager and not eager enough. It will probably test your patience too. But this I can promise you; once he has let you have your way, and you have shown how good you are at it, he will never protest again. Men who have never experienced being made love to by an expert woman can never know what a thrilling experience it can be.

I am sure I do not have to point out, however, that you will have to be good to make him really appreciate you. It is no good your going to great lengths to get your way, if at the end of it you do not put up a really first-class performance. So before you make your proposal make absolutely certain that you have discovered all his sensitive zones and the type of caress which draws most response from each one; the combination of sensitive zones which, caressed simultaneously, most turn him on; and the length of time he usually takes when he starts from scratch and is taking the active role. If you go on much longer than he usually takes himself, you will probably put him off.

When you make love to him he should lie on his back, because this exposes to you the majority of his sensitive zones. At the same time, however, don't neglect his back. At one point during loveplay, get him to turn over on to his tummy, then reclining beside him, run the tip of your tongue lightly down the length of his spine, beginning at the nape of his neck and going down to the beginning of the cleft of his buttock. Stroke his buttocks lightly with a hand, or knead them with both hands. Whichever you know thrills him most.

Two sensitive zones are nearly always overlooked—a man's nipples and his perineum, the ridge which runs from his anal opening up behind his scrotum to the base of his penis. The nipples are overlooked because a man's nipples, unlike a woman's, are not connected by nerves to his sexual nervous system. Many men are quite unaware themselves that despite this apparent lack of connection their nipples may be highly responsive to sucking or rolling between finger and thumb, in the same way that a woman's nipples are. Mind you, not all men's nipples are responsive, though many more are than the men themselves realize. Some are so responsive that many younger men can not only bring on erection but bring themselves to orgasm—or be brought to orgasm—by stimulation of the nipples alone. If your man has prominent nipples, there is an eight to two chance that they will be sensitive.

The perineum is overlooked, by both men and women—women have one, too, from the anal opening to the vaginal entrance—because it is rather hidden away. You should be able to feel the muscle which surrounds the basis of the penis, when the man voluntarily or involuntarily twitches it. If you press on this muscle at the midpoint of the perineum you can induce an erection if the penis is limp, or make the erection stronger if it is rather weak. The best way of stimulating the perineum is with the tongue. Get your partner to lie across the bed with his buttocks as near to the edge of the bed as possible, with his knees drawn up and the sides of his feet on the bed. Kneel by the bed, and beginning with the end of the perineum nearer the anus, run the tip of the tongue slowly up it, up over the scrotum, up the penis shaft, to the head, pause for a moment or two to tease the frenum and penis tip with the tip of the tongue, then take the tongue back the way it has come to the perineum.

But people like myself can go on making suggestions of this kind until the cows come home, when nothing that we can suggest can really match what you discover for yourself by experimenting and exploring. Range wide, because you never know whether your partner may not have some special *personal* sensitive zone, which he may never know about unless you find it for him. We are all such individuals in our responses to sex that only by treating each other as a special case can we ever hope fully to realize ourselves sexually.

So remember: If you accept, as I sincerely hope you do, that lovemaking, as a reflection of the marriage relationship as a whole, is an *equal* partnership with *equal* responsibilities for each partner, then you must, by the very nature of lovemaking, be an active partner. Above all, you must not restrict your activity to those occasions when you are taking the active role from initiation to orgasm, but every time you and your partner make love. If you do accept these ideas, then I can assure you, your lovemaking should leave nothing to be desired.

Chapter NINE

"My Husband Has Been Unfaithful"

One good thing I hope the new British divorce law will do is to impress upon people that one, two, or even three acts of adultery need not break up a marriage. In the past couples have rushed all too eagerly to the lawyers without pausing to think what may have been the cause for the spouse's infidelity, because in 95 cases out of 100 there is a specific cause, even if it is only a spontaneous act committed because the opportunity presented itself. Men are more prone to this kind of thoughtless infidelity than women, because, like it or not, the man's whole concept of the significance of lovemaking is quite different from the woman's. Let me enlarge on this a little, because, in my view, it is necessary that women should understand this.

All tied up with the mother instinct, the carrying of the baby in the womb, and the former concept of the significance of virginity—once her vagina has been penetrated by a penis the woman can never be the same as she was before; she has lost something (her hymen)—the woman's whole approach to physical lovemaking is basically much more meaningful to her than the man's is to him. Unless she is seeking only the physical sensations of lovemaking the woman always becomes emotionally involved to some extent. In actual fact, when I advocate that physical lovemaking should be used to express the emotional love the couple have for one another, as far as the woman is concerned I am preaching to the already converted, though most women do not realize it.

Men can make love without emotional involvement. They will have an affection for the partner and be kind to her and appreciative of her, but half an hour later, unless he has fallen in love with her, the man can forget her.

You must not blame him for this; it is how he is made. It comes from the basic difference between the man's much more rapid response to stimulation and the ease with which he comes and the woman's equivalent but much, much slower responses; and to the fact that after he has ejaculated his semen into her, he has played his part, while she, if she conceives, goes on playing her part for another two hundred and eighty days.

Women must understand this difference, and not be hurt by it. They need not be hurt by it and may never have cause to be, because when a man becomes emotionally involved with a woman, i.e., falls in love with her, there is little to choose between the qualities of the two kinds of loving. Yet I would not be wholly honest if I did not admit that even when a man deeply loves a woman, he can, if the opportunity presents itself and the mood is right, pop into bed with another woman without considering whether he is rocking the boat insofar as his marriage relationship is concerned. It is his own reactions afterwards which can play a bit of havoc, but usually he can pass even them over, if he can assure himself that nothing has happened to interfere with his relationship with his wife.

But, please, don't let me give you the wrong impression. If a man's marriage relationship is sound and his sexual relationship a happy one, he is most unlikely to try his sexual luck elsewhere. He won't have a reason to. If he does, it will be on the spur of the moment, and will mean little or nothing to him.

Still, the question remains, and it is a very important one: How much infidelity should a marriage take, can a marriage take? Let us consider one or two of the more usual types of case.

Lydia had been married to Alfred for five years when she discovered he was being unfaithful. When she tackled him with it, he admitted it, but promised to be good in future if she would forgive him this once. He kept his word for nearly a year.

Lydia then discovered his second affair. Her first reaction was to leave him, but when she calmed down, she decided not to seek a divorce for the sake of the children. However, she did tell Alfred she knew, and again he promised to be good. For some time she had no reason to doubt that he was keeping his word. Then, when the oldest child, a boy, was seventeen, and the youngest, a girl, thirteen, once more she found out that Alfred was having another affair.

When she accused him, he laughed and confessed.

"But why?" she asked.

"I like this girl," he said. "She's fun and—well, I like going to bed with her."

"Don't I mean anything to you any more?"

"Of course you do. You're the mother of my children and you look after me very well."

"Don't you love me any more, then?"

"Do you love me? Be honest! The trouble is we've got used to one another, and I don't mind admitting our lovemaking bores me."

"But why didn't you say so. I would have done my best to please you. I've never refused you, have I? Or to do anything you wanted me to do?"

"Haven't you? You may not have said anything, but you've made it plain in other ways that you're not all that interested in sex."

"But you should have told me."

"Anyway, it's too late now. We're too old to pick up the threads again, so what do you want to do?"

"I'll have to think about it," she said.

David swept Clare off her feet with his whirlwind wooing. He made love to her the fourth time they met, and a day or two later asked her to marry him. She accepted and within two months they were married, despite friends' and parents' warnings of the disaster for which they might be heading. David was generous, appreciative, loving, always good-humored. As a lover he was superb. He was proud of her and enjoyed showing her off to his friends. In the face of her happiness and David's, friends and relations admitted they had been wrong.

In connection with his business, David traveled a good deal, though he was rarely away for more than two nights at a time. Clare discovered that he was being unfaithful to her when, turning out the pockets of a suit before sending it to the cleaners, she came upon an old diary. In the back of the diary was a list of girls' names and telephone numbers, and the names of all appeared under various dates throughout the diary. Also in the suit was a letter from a girl which left no doubt that she and David had recently made love.

Clare's first reaction was to pack her bags and leave home. But the thought that if she did it would prove her parents and relations right after all, made her pause. David was away until the following day; she would think it over, she decided.

By the time David was due home, she had made up her mind to confront him and threaten that if ever again she discovered he was being unfaithful, she would divorce him.

"As soon as he opened the door and held out his arms to me," she told me, "I forgot everything I was going to say. All the warmth that had fled from the house the moment I found that beastly diary and letter came into the room with him. There could be no possibility at all of his not loving me, and if he loved me, he couldn't love anyone else. What did it matter, then, who he took to bed for an hour or two? So long as I was sure that he still loved me, I would be a fool to be jealous of what he might be doing with any other woman, that is, provided he was discreet about it.

"He must have been because I never had any hint of them. Mind you, I think he knew I knew, because I left the diary and letter on his dressing table. He didn't say anything, but he did go a bit pale when he saw them. Knowing his nature, however, I suspect he hasn't changed. We're still as happy as the day we married. The serious rows we've had you could count on the fingers of one hand."

Robert S was posted overseas in 1942. A few months later he was taken prisoner of war. He was released and returned home in 1945.

While he had been away, his wife, Marian, joined the WAAF and had two or three casual affairs with officers on her station. She became pregnant as a result of one of these, but her lover procured an abortion for her.

She did not apply for demobilization immediately on Robert's return, and he was given permission to join her on her station for a time, as they had no home. It did not take him long to discover that shortly before his arrival, she had embarked on another affair. When he asked her about it, she freely admitted it, and wishing to wipe her slate clean, she told him everything, including the abortion.

Maybe it was too much for his still upset state of mind to consider calmly. Had he been able to pause and think, it is more than likely that he would have appreciated the situation in which Marian had found herself. She was an extremely attractive young woman, separated from her husband by the artificial circumstances of war, and thrown among a number of young men who risked their lives every day, and who longed for a few moments of intimacy to shut out the ever-present horrors. Marian, too, missed the comfort of love and the security of Robert's arms about her. One might say that being what they were, where they were, human nature would have been very inept indeed if it had not brought her and the young men together, so that each might give the other brief periods of solace.

Robert did not see it like that. He packed his bag and went to his parents' home, determined to have nothing more to do with Marian. Fortunately, he did not take immediate action. He did not even take his parents into his confidence, and his mother put his moodiness down to his POW experiences.

A few days after he arrived home, while brooding over it all, he suddenly realized that he still loved Marian, and pursuing this train of thought, it occurred to him, "If I opt out now it's as good as admitting that I'm inferior to this fellow." This he could not accept. To prove himself better than Marian's lover was, he would get her away from him, get her back.

He told me, "I wrote asking her to get a few days' leave, or at least a seventy-two-hour pass, if she could, and we would go away somewhere by ourselves and talk things over. We didn't talk long. When we were alone, I said to her, 'Let's forget all about these last years and carry on from where we stopped, shall we?' 'Yes, please,' she said, and we clung to one another and cried a bit and then made love, and it was better than it had ever been. That was twenty-three years ago, and I don't think any couple have been happier than we've been, and still are. I've never even thought about what Marian told me, unless I've been specially reminded. I've forgotten more than half of it, any way. If I do think about it, it is to tell myself that Marian wasn't to blame for anything."

Isabel had been brought up against a puritanical home background, by a mother who thought all sex was disgusting. She was twenty-six when she married Harry, who was five years older.

"Why I was attracted to her, I've no idea," Harry was to tell me twelve years later. "I was—still am—very fond of sex, and need a go at least once a day. When I first made a pass at her, a simple caress of a breast over her dress, she pushed my hand away angrily, saying she didn't like playing around, it was dirty. But she could be fun to be with, and I knew she would be a good housekeeper from the way she managed her own finances.

"I discovered what I had let myself in for sex-wise within a few months of getting married. She wouldn't undress if I was in the room. She bought me pajamas because she thought sleeping raw was disgusting. I knew she wasn't experienced, so I tried to teach her, breaking her in gently after the first three months. Well, to cut a long story short, we've been married twelve years and in all that time she's never let me do more than play with a nipple and finger her clitoris; she's never done anything to me but hold my cock for a minute or two. Only twice have we used the woman-above position and that's the only other position we have used besides the missionary position. I tried to go down on her once and she went and slept in the spare room, and when I was mad enough to ask her to do a blow-job on me—only asked, mind you—she didn't speak to me for a week.

"You can imagine how frustrating this has been for a chap like me who really loves his oats. I don't see how anyone can blame me for getting a bit on the side whenever I can. If it hadn't been for the children, I would have asked for a divorce, though I'm sure she wouldn't have given me one because of what the family and neighbors might say. For the last four years I've had a permanent mistress who wants it as much as I do, and doesn't mind what she does so long as it's pleasant. If it hadn't been for her, I'd have gone crazy with frustration long ago."

These case histories, which I have extracted at random from my files, demonstrate the traditional main causes for men and women committing adultery: boredom, compulsive promiscuousness, enforced long periods of separation, and the refusal of one partner to meet even halfway the sexual needs of the other, by cooperating in techniques of lovemaking that will satisfy these needs. There is also one other main cause—neglect, which, our social structure being what it is, more often leads the wife astray than the husband.

Frank L was in his late forties. He had been married to Joan for twenty years, and they had a boy aged nineteen and a girl of seventeen.

For the past ten years Frank had been completely

wrapped up in his job. During the first five he had worked to fulfill his ambition to become managing director; during the second five, he worked to make himself the best managing director his firm had ever had. In the process his home became for him little more than a hotel, and his wife merely his housekeeper. True, they shared a bedroom still, but if they made love half a dozen times a year, Joan regarded it as something of a miracle.

Joan, some seven years younger, was approaching middle age with a maturing beauty which made many of her women friends envious. She took care of her figure and complexion, and dressed well. Despite her attempts to understand what made Frank tick, there were many occasions when she felt the absence of love acutely.

One day her car broke down on a lonely stretch of road. A motorist stopped, examined the engine without success, and promised to get assistance from the first garage he came to. When the tow truck arrived, Joan was surprised to see the man following in his car.

"I thought I'd come back." He smiled. "It struck me it might be serious and you wouldn't be able to get home."

His surmise had been right. The car needed a major repair. He drove Joan to the garage, waited while she completed the formalities, and then drove her home. On the way home they exchanged names and one or two other items of personal information. Though she judged him to be between thirty-five and forty, he was unmarried, Joan discovered, and a stockbroker. He was good-looking, dressed well, had dark brown eyes that twinkled with laughter all the time, and his voice was deep and resonant.

Joan thanked him for his kindness when he dropped her off at the house. He hoped they would meet again, and Joan said she hoped so, too, though she secretly supposed they would not. She was wrong, however. Three days later, he called her and asked her to dine. As Frank was away on business, she accepted.

They dined in a discreet restaurant and were quietly happy. Under the influence of his attentions, Joan glowed with long-forgotten pleasure. When he took her home, she asked him in for a drink, and before he left they made love, in a way Joan had never realized love could be made. Next morning Joan was horrified by what she had done, and determined never to let it happen again.

When he telephoned a few days later, she explained how she felt. He persuaded her to see him just once more.

"MY HUSBAND HAS BEEN UNFAITHFUL" 109

She agreed reluctantly, and they made love a second time. This time Joan was not so horrified by what she had done, and from then on they met whenever they could.

In my view, three of the reasons I have illustrated justify adultery—neglect, enforced long separation, and the refusal to cooperate or even meet the other partner halfway in lovemaking. Compulsive promiscuousness I also have to recognize as justifiable, with the proviso that the compulsive adulterer or adulteress takes the greatest care to keep his adultery completely hidden from the partner so that the partner is not hurt. Only boredom do I find to be a completely invalid reason.

The main point about adultery is that in all but the most exceptional cases, the faithful partner stands to get hurt. There is no more cruel sex crime, in my opinion, than making it apparent to the partner that he/she is inadequate to satisfy one's sexual needs. There are very, very few women—or men—like Clare, who have the wisdom to see that compulsive promiscuousness is not the result of dissatisfaction with the marital sex life.

So far as I can discover, no serious research has yet been carried out into why the compulsive adulterer behaves as he does. The ones I have met have been pleasant enough men and women, highly sexed, in no other way immoral, but in this particular behavior unable to see that they may be behaving immorally and can be hurtful. "But," they say, "we don't love our casual partners. We reserve love for our wives."

I put it to one compulsive adulterer that even if the wife were not hurt, the casual partner might be.

"I can't speak for others," he said, "but I am absolutely honest with my casual partners. I always tell them that I'm married. . . ."

"But that your wife doesn't understand you?" I suggested.

"On the contrary, I tell them that my wife loves me and I love her, and that we are very happy sexually and otherwise. They come to bed with me of their own free choice, in the full knowledge that I will never marry one of them. I don't want to sound boastful, but I think they know before the first time, that I shall be good in bed. I've never yet had a partner who hasn't been as sexually uninhibited as I am. Why, I can't think. We just set out to give one another the best time we can, and that creates a bond between us which isn't love, but it gives our fucking a reason and a dignity which prevents it from being an expression of shameless lust."

In the cases I have known where neglect was the cause of the adultery, it has always been the woman who has been neglected. Nearly all have led to discovery and divorce, for the same sort of reasons that Frank L divorced Joan.

Frank overheard Joan making an assignation with her lover over the extension telephone. He said nothing to Joan, but next day arranged for a private detective to watch her. As a result of the detective's report, he filed a petition for divorce, citing the stockbroker. Joan knew nothing of his intentions until the petition was served on her.

By this time Joan had had another heart-searching and had decided she must put a stop to these pleasant interludes, though they had completely transformed her life. She promised Frank that if he would withdraw the petition she would never again be unfaithful. She pointed out that her affair had lasted only five weeks, and that she and her lover had been to bed fewer than a dozen times. Frank refused to listen.

Asked why he could not forgive Joan for this single lapse, Frank replied, "How do I know it won't happen again? Anyway, how can I go on living with her after she has done this, in spite of all I've done for her. I've never been unfaithful to her, and I've given her everything she's asked for. Besides, if anyone else found out they wouldn't think much of me if I didn't take action. I daren't risk that."

In other words, he would not apply the solution he had in his own hands—devoting some time in and out of bed to Joan. He was much more prepared to sacrifice his marriage to preserve his business reputation; in other words, he was more prepared to apply his ruthless business code to his family life, purely so that in the eyes of his business colleagues he should remain above reproach.

When adultery by either party occurs as the result of long periods of separation, I feel it is a part of the human experience which ought to be accepted by both, and ignored. For both husband and wife who have known the consolation of physical intimacy it should be taken more as a compliment than an insult if either or both try to recapture the joy and contentment in someone else's arms because they miss it so. I believe that most couples who are in this category—and all I know are people who are deeply in love—do appreciate this, for one rarely meets with a case which ends in divorce.

In my view, the most justifiable adultery of all results from the refusal of a partner to recognize and try to supply the sexual needs of the other. Unlike the case I have quoted, in most cases when this happens, with the wonderful perverseness of human nature, the adulterous partner continues to love and respect the uncooperative partner. If the adulterous relationship is conducted with the utmost discretion, so that the uncooperative partner remains in his/her rosy glow of ignorance, then the role of the mistress or lover assumes commendable proportions. Many a marriage has been preserved by a mistress or lover who has provided the sexual comfort that the partner has been unable to provide.

Adultery committed out of boredom I have absolutely to condemn. It need not happen and should not happen. Both partners are specifically to blame for allowing boredom to overtake their sex life. I need not go into the details of the remedy here; put briefly, variety in lovemaking, imaginative lovemaking, and constant experimenting with techniques keep boredom at bay. But it is most often the man who commits adultery in boredom cases, and I have no sympathy whatsoever for him, because he is so sex-lazy that rather than reinvigorate his marital relationship he seeks a cure for his boredom in variety, usually choosing partners who, of their own volition, are "fun in bed," so that he shall not be required to exert himself sexually-imaginatively.

Boredom-adultery cases, perhaps inevitably, drift, unless the faithful partner is of strong character. After a number of challenges and a number of threats, the adulterer becomes case-hardened. The third time Lydia challenged Alfred, he did not ask for forgiveness. He would have been upset if she had taken action, but only because he would have had a comfortable way of life disrupted. But he was pretty certain she would not take action, and she did not. She could not face the unpleasantness which even the innocent party in a divorce has to face from family and friends, however much they may seem to sympathize. So she let things drift.

"I know I'm a moral coward," she said, "but I just couldn't go through with it. I made up my mind to live with it, because I knew I couldn't do anything else."

Couldn't or wouldn't? When she said that, she was thirty-eight years old. She had another lifetime of boredom and misery before her, unless as she grew older, she became bolder.

It is my view that no couple need be bored in bed and that they would not be bored if they shed all their inhibitions and set about making themselves truly proficient lovers. With all the books, films and other sources of information that are now available, plus the couple's own inventive powers, the permutations that can be devised are infinite.

Then there are mechanical aids—vibrators, contoured sheaths, clitoral stimulators and vaginal stimulators and other ingenious devices—easily obtainable, by mail order (under plain cover) or over the counter in many of the big cities—not all of them, of course. No couple, who feel that they have tried everything and can think of nothing more, should hesitate to coopt these toys. The use of anything that will heighten and so enrich the sexual experience is fully justified, though I do think that the use of aids should be a last resort, since their fitting on and the knowledge that they are present can take away much of the spontaneity which I believe is essential for successful love-expressive lovemaking.

It is nowadays argued by sex-bored couples that one of the most effective cures is permissive adultery in an exchange of partners. I have reservations, however, about the ultimate wisdom and efficaciousness of wife-swapping, whether between two couples in the privacy of their own homes or at parties where a draw, by car keys or other personal objects, is made to select random partners. With regard to the latter, there has to be some rapport between sexual partners, for without some psychological response the physical response is doomed to be low-grade. This is particularly true of women.

But the real danger of both the private two-couple or three-couple groups and of the multi-couple-random-partner group is that once the exchange has been made, the couples go to separate rooms and make love in solitude. I have only taken part in such an experiment once, some years before the last war, when we had reached a crisis in our relationship, and instead of it effecting a cure, only a miracle saved our marriage from breaking up. (This was the experience of our partners, too.) Because we knew that the other was making love in the next bedroom, we could not concentrate on our own lovemaking.

"MY HUSBAND HAS BEEN UNFAITHFUL" 113

What were the other two doing? Was J enjoying it? Would she enjoy it more than she did with me? Would it be so good that she would forever afterwards taunt me with the high competence of Paul as a lover compared with my own mediocre skills? Whenever we made love, would she wish it was Paul and not me? Even if we made up our differences, would Paul ever be forgotten?

Suspicion and jealousy and fear were our dominant reactions, and I have talked to other couples who have tried the experiment and whose reactions have tallied with ours. I know there are many couples who claim just the reverse, but I have never yet personally met one such couple, who, put on their honor, insisted that it had enhanced their physical relationship with their spouses. It might have dispelled their boredom, but their experience was no richer on that account. And there have been many couples whose exchange of partners has led directly to the divorce courts.

It was suspicion that was the main cause of our failure, and I think that if, after we had made the exchange, all of us had made love in the same room, so that we could have checked visually occasionally what was happening to the partner, we might have been more successful.

Group sex, which many confuse with wife-swapping, can be very helpful, in my opinion, if taken part in occasionally. Everyone of us is voyeur enough to be highly stimulated by the sight of the lovemaking of others, and the memories of it can be used to great advantage in enhancing one's own lovemaking at home. It is not always required that one should exchange partners, but if one wishes to do so, the exchanges need not be made until one has found someone with whom one has some measure of rapport. If this rapport does not make itself apparent, then, in my view, no exchange should be made.

Since one can, during group sex, keep an eye on the partner's activities, suspicion and jealousy are unlikely to arise, and finally there is the considerable practical advantage that by watching others making love, one almost invariably picks up a new hint or two. Knowing, too, that one is also probably being watched, puts one on one's mettle, so that one pulls out all the stops to provide the best performance possible. This effort has a long-term effect on the marital sex scene which can be exactly the boost the relationship needs.

The new British divorce law, which makes the irretrievable breakdown of marriage the only grounds on which a decree can be obtained, has been called the adulterer's charter. I do not see this. Persistent adultery on the part of either partner can still cause a marriage to break up. As I said at the beginning, however, one good thing I hope it will do, is to make people think again, both carefully and long, before rushing to the courts. But even this cannot change the nature of adultery, which, in my view, can never be a prophylactic against sex-boredom or sex-laziness, the two most prevalent causes of extramarital sex.

Chapter TEN

"My Husband Has Problems"

When a woman writes this to me, more often than not she is referring not to some shortcoming in her partner's sexual performance or capacity, but to his strange requests, outside the ordinary run of lovemaking techniques, or to his strange behavior either inside or outside the marriage relationship. Nearly always what is known as a deviation is involved, and because to many this word has frightening attributes, such cries for help need special consideration.

What is sexual deviation, or as it was formerly termed, *perversion*, all about?

To make the subject as simple as possible, let us talk about just one aspect of our lives—our social behavior. Society has laid down certain rules for our behavior in public. It requires us, for example, to conduct ourselves in an orderly fashion, not to go pushing people out of the way in order to do or get what we want to do or get; not to go about in public places with our genitals uncovered; not to urinate in public, not to break certain rules specific to certain places, e.g., commercial vehicles are not allowed in certain places at certain times; and so on. There is laid down for us, in other words, a code of general and particular rules of behavior, aimed at making the ordinary everyday conduct and movement of individuals the least upsetting to the majority. Without such a code of conduct there would be absolute chaos.

As with every other aspect of our behavioral existence there are certain standards of behavior in our sexual activities. These standards are based on the behavior patterns of the majority, and without such standards it would be impossible to comment upon sexual behavior. The chief of these standards is penis-vagina contact as the termination of lovemaking, the means of achieving orgasm in both partners and ejaculation in the male. Any other means of achieving sexual satisfaction deviates from this norm, or standard.

Unfortunately, the words perversion and deviation, which are used to label departures from the norm, are applied to any and every such departure. They are also words which are highly charged with emotions, the pervert (or deviate) being regarded by most "straight" men and women as someone not nice to know. But as with everything else, there are many degrees of difference in deviation. Let me try to give a few examples.

Probably the best known deviations are sadism and masochism. The sadist can only achieve full sexual satisfaction if he/she inflicts physical pain on the partner; the masochist only if pain is inflicted on him/her. (Though this sounds a terrible way of obtaining satisfaction, and many lurid accounts of what sadists do to their victims and what masochists beg to have done to them come to notice nearly every day—whipping, binding in chains, and so on—it is very, very rare that the sadist does his victim physical harm or the masochist needs beatings and tortures of such ferocity that he is physically harmed.) Besides being the best known deviations, sadism and masochism also raise a great deal of emotional opposition, chiefly, I think, because we are very preoccupied in these days with violence in films and on television and in certain kinds of books, but also because cruelty is considered to be alien to the intelligence of the human mind and to the human character. But there are many other deviations only by the practice of which can the sufferers obtain sexual satisfaction, that are far more disgusting than sadism and masochism, for example, intercourse with animals, coprophilia (which is an abnormal interest in urine and feces, sometimes accompanied by the desire to drink and eat them, though usually to have them deposited on the body), gerontophilia (sexual intercourse between a young man and a very old woman) or necrophilia (the use of a dead body as a sexual object). Because these are much less frequently heard of, they tend to be outside the knowledge of the man in the street, but this does not mean to say they occur less frequently (with the possible exception of necrophilia) than sadism and masochism.

But now let us look at another deviation. The normal way of obtaining orgasm is by penis-vagina contact. Occasionally a couple will use oral lovemaking or mutual masturbation right through to orgasm to obtain their satisfaction. If they obtain satisfaction in this way less frequently than they do by penis-vagina contact then they are not practicing a deviation. However, some couples develop a preference for oral intercourse and *always* obtain orgasm through it, or use it far more frequently than they do penis-vagina contact. When this happens they have become deviants. But the permanent use of oral intercourse or mutual masturbation cannot cause either partner any physical harm, it is not an activity involving any degree of cruelty, unless one partner is forced to do it against his/her will, and it has neither disgusting nor bestial features like coprophilia, necrophilia, and bestiality. There is, therefore, a great deal of difference between real lovemaking as a deviation and, say, sadism and masochism.

It is customary for the entirely normally sexual person to regard the deviant as an inferior human being who ought not to be accepted in decent society. But is this point of view justified? I don't think it is!

Over and over again, when talking about lovemaking techniques in answer to questions such as "Is cunnilingus or fellatio normal?" "Is rear-entry normal?" or, "Is making love in the bath normal?" I repeat, *there is nothing that a man and woman can do with one another sexually in the privacy of their home, that can be degrading, immoral or sinful provided that neither party is forced to carry out any act against his/her will and is, therefore, not hurt by it physically or psychologically*. In my view this cardinal rule of all sexual behavior is as applicable to couples practicing deviations as it is to any other technique of loveplay, because when all is said and done, the majority of deviant practices are loveplay techniques.

It is in connection with mild forms of deviation in their partner's sexual behavior that most women write to me. The more extreme deviators do not seem to want help. No research has been done on this subject so far, but the sadists who go the whole way seem to have the ability to find masochistic partners, which is the ideal partnership for them, while the coprophiliacs and the gerontophiliacs very rarely reveal their preferences more widely than to partners whom they either persuade to cooperate or lose before they have finished explaining what they want of them.

I think most people, men and women, who have no abnormal desires themselves, shy away when they first come into contact with deviant desires. While it is in part natural that they should react in this way, it is, in my view, chiefly ignorance of why some people cannot gain sexual satisfaction in the normal way, ignorance of exactly what the deviant behavior consists of, and the result of the exaggerated views of most deviations that have been extremely widespread in most western cultures for centuries.

There are a good many mild deviations, however, which scarcely merit the name. For example, spanking.

Dear Mr. Chartham: I am very worried about my husband and hope you will be able to help me. I am twenty-five and he is twenty-seven and we have been married about eighteen months. I love him dearly and if I read the signs aright, he loves me as much. He is a skillful lover, kind and considerate, and I enjoy our lovemaking tremendously. In fact, I have always done so. So why am I writing to you?

Well, a few months ago he asked me to spank his bottom with an ordinary flat twelve-inch ruler while we were making love. I have no sadistic tendencies; in fact, I'm just the opposite. The idea of even hurting a small animal unintentionally upsets me, and the thought of inflicting pain on my husband I find equally upsetting. I've explained all this to him, but he still keeps asking me, and lately begged me to spank him. He got so nervous one night about two weeks ago that very reluctantly I did what he asked, I didn't hit him very hard, but his buttocks became quite red, and the redder they became the more he squirmed in the way one does when experiencing great physical pleasure. He breathed very hard and kept making quiet exclamations. He was lying on his tummy, and as he got really worked up he began to thrust with his buttocks against the bed, just as he does when he is in me, and after a moment or two he gave a gasp, and a shudder shook him from head to foot, and then he lay still. I knew what had happened, of course, and didn't know what to do next.

After a moment or two, he turned to me. His reaction was quite puzzling—a kind of gratitude mixed with shame. He kept thanking me and then saying how sorry he was that he had come. But after a few minutes, he began to make love to me, and, if anything, the session was even more passionate than our lovemaking usually is.

I was worried because I didn't understand it, and I

"MY HUSBAND HAS PROBLEMS" 119

was grateful when he did not ask me to do it again until last night. I sort of sensed that he was going to ask me as we got ready for bed, and that made me nervous. But funnily enough, when he asked me, I didn't hesitate. Much the same thing happened as on the previous occasion, except that toward the end, he seized me rather roughly, came into me and came with a terrific orgasm, and then made me come. Again he thanked me, and kept telling me what a wonderful girl I was.

Now that I have done it and seen what pleasure it gives him, though I wouldn't do it unless he asked me, I don't mind doing it for him occasionally. But what I am afraid of is that he will want me to do it more often and progressively harder, so that the time will arrive when he won't be able to come without my beating him quite hard. When I realized that he was masochistic I asked myself whether I would have married him had I known. My first reaction was, no, I wouldn't. But now I'm not so sure. He is such a wonderful husband and such a kind man, that I think I would have said yes. In fact, I'm sure I would.

But I am honestly worried about what to do for the best. Ought I to spank him when he asks me to, or am I encouraging him to become a real masochist? Will it affect him in the opposite direction if I refuse? What do you advise?

P.S. What can have caused him to have this "kink?"

My first reaction to this letter was, "Thank goodness for a sensible, intelligent girl!" This is what I replied to her.

Your husband's "kink," as you call it, is much more common than is, I think, generally supposed. Its beginnings can usually be traced back to a childhood incident at school, and as corporal punishment in English schools, especially boys' public schools, used to be—and still is in some schools—quite a common practice, Englishmen seem to be more prone to wanting to be spanked, than boys in other countries where beatings are not a punishment, or are used only rarely.

The relationship between physical pain and sexual arousal is a very complicated subject, and it has not been thoroughly explored yet. Though it is more than likely he has forgotten all about it, he will probably have had a beating at school during which he experienced erection and orgasm. It may have been a result of a first beating or a subsequent one, but somehow the connection between pain and sexual arousal made an impact on his subconscious, and to eradicate it now would probably take a long course of psychotherapy. The thing to consider is, would such a treatment be justified?

I shall be very surprised indeed if his masochistic tendencies become more extreme as time goes by. The chief point to be considered, I suggest, is your own attitude toward it. If you really don't mind doing it for him, there is no reason why you shouldn't. The chances of your developing sadistic tendencies are practically nil. One thing I think you ought not to do is to spank him every time you make love. Obviously that is what he would like you to do, but as he does seem to be able to get some measure of sexual satisfaction without being spanked; and since you are only agreeing to spank him because you love him and it makes him happy, and don't get any enjoyment out of it yourself, then, to my mind, he ought to forgo this special pleasure sometimes as a *quid pro quo* for your cooperation. I suggest you discuss it with him. Tell him exactly what you feel about it; if you agree with the suggestion I have just made, put that to him; see what he has to say; and then reach a compromise between you.

I can't tell you how wise you have been in overcoming your reluctance to the extent of being able to do what he wants. This is where so many wives make such a bad mistake, not in this kind of case, but in what I suppose one must call "advanced" lovemaking techniques. They have been so conditioned psychologically, or religiously, to what is "normal" sex—which doesn't really exist—that they not only cannot but *will not* compromise or cooperate. You see, what one could almost guarantee happening in your case is this: If you adamantly refuse to cooperate with your husband's little sexual whim (because that is what it really amounts to; his masochistic tendencies, though present, are not at all extreme; he doesn't want to be tied up, gagged and assaulted, or made to grovel, or go about on all fours with a dog-collar round his neck, and led by you on a chain) sooner or later his failure to fulfill his desires will mount up into quite a sizable frustration.

Eventually the time will come when his frustration will be absolutely unbearable and then two things are likely to happen; he will turn against you and your marriage will fall apart, and he will find another woman, in any case, who will supply his particular sexual need. The more he bottles it up, the worse the crash will be when it comes. (If I may suggest it, you must give him some credit for having the courage to seek your cooperation. Equally many husbands make the mistake of keeping their more advanced desires from their wives, with identical eventual results, and in many cases, totally needlessly, since many of the wives would have cooperated if asked.)

All this can be avoided by your cooperation. In fact, I feel certain that as a result of your cooperation, you will find your relationship becoming deeper and more satisfying, not merely in the sexual sphere, than it could otherwise have become. Think over what I have suggested, and above all talk to your husband about it!

Don't hesitate to write to me again if you feel I can help any further in any way.

(She wrote to me about a week later thanking me, and telling me that they had discussed the difficulty frankly and completely, and had arrived at a very happy and satisfying sexual way of life.)

There are other little sexual quirks which can be accepted by a woman if only she will realize that they have no far-reaching consequences unless they are completely frustrated. Not long ago, a woman wrote to me that after sixteen years of happy and satisfying love life, her husband had become impotent. (He was partially impotent, as a matter of fact, because he could get an erection under certain circumstances, it eventually transpired.) It had upset him as much as it had her, but try as they might, they could do nothing which would help restore his erection during lovemaking. One night, in their mutual frustration, they lost their tempers with one another and during a rather terrifying row, the husband, not realizing what he was saying, blurted out, "It would all be all right, if only you . . ."

What he wants me to do [she wrote] is to parade up and down the bedroom in front of him naked except for a black nylon girdle which had a circle cut out of the middle so that my naval will be exposed. Has he gone mad? Is there any cure? Am I really saddled with a pervert?

As they lived in London I asked her to come and see me. I let her let rip about her husband and his quaint desire (though the quaintness in no way lessened the importance of its fulfillment). When she had run out of words, and ideas, and finished with, "Is there any cure?" I told her that although psychotherapy might cure him, there was a much simpler way of remedying the wretched situation in which they found themselves. If she would get herself a black nylon girdle and cut out the bit that covered her navel and then walked up and down the bedroom for a few minutes her husband's potency would almost certainly be restored.

"But I couldn't do that!" she exclaimed.

"Why not?"

"I'd feel such a fool."

"And is your feeling a fool or not feeling a fool more important to you than your sex life and your marriage? Don't you love your husband enough to do this little unimportant thing for him? Do you want your marriage to break up? Do you want to go through the rest of your life without making love, that is, unless you divorce? I don't see why you should feel a fool when you are doing it for your husband, and no one else will ever know but the two of you."

"But it will be encouraging him in his kinkiness!"

"So what?" I said. "So long as it doesn't hurt you, or degrade you in his eyes—and it won't—it's a pretty harmless kink, and I honestly can't see why you shouldn't encourage him in it when you can both benefit so much by encouraging him."

We said a good deal more to one another, but before she left I got her to promise to think over seriously what I had suggested. Apparently she thought it over without loss of time, because four or five days later I had this letter.

After leaving you, on the way home I stopped and bought a black nylon girdle and before J came home I cut a piece out of the middle. I went up to bed some time before J, got undressed, put on the girdle and a bed-jacket and got in bed to read. I nearly fell asleep and ruined it all before J eventually came up, but when he had got into bed, and we'd said goodnight—we don't even kiss now—I slipped out of bed and took off the bed-jacket and began to sidle up and down the bedroom. I must admit I felt a bit of a fool, but then a funny thing happened. J began to snore, and that struck me as very funny ha-ha and I burst out laughing and woke him up. "What the hell's amusing you," he said, "what are you standing there for?" Then he saw me properly and shot up in bed, and a smile spread slowly over his face, such a kind and grateful smile, and he sort of half-whispered, "Oh, A." Well, I paraded around for a moment, not a bit self-conscious any more, until after a minute or two he said, "Take that thing off and come to bed now!" So I did, and when I touched him he was as stiff as a poker. I just couldn't believe it, and had to look to make sure he wasn't pulling a fast one. But he wasn't, and we had one of the best fucks we'd had for years. It happened again the next night and the next; and last night he got an erection without me having to do anything. All of a sudden life has changed from hell to paradise. He's so appreciative. He came home with a lovely piece of jewelry for me the day before yesterday, something he hasn't done for ages. I don't know how to thank you for making me see that feeling a fool—I don't any longer, anyway—was of far less importance than making J, and myself, happy.

The husband's special wish in this case did not really amount to a fetish, but fetishism does come into married life quite often, and again can raise all kinds of misgivings in the wife's mind. Again, most fetishes are absolutely harmless, and the wise and loving wife will not object to them. As with other deviations, ignorance of what fetishism really is causes more than half the trouble.

First of all, 99.9 percent, possibly more, of all fetishists are men. Briefly and simply, when a man becomes a fetishist, his sexual desire (libido) becomes fixated on a lifeless symbol which represents the love-object for him. The objects chosen cover a very wide range. Hair from the head and pubic hair, women's panties, furs, high-heeled shoes, women's gloves, rubber garments, leather jackets, leather boots, and so on, as well as some more strange objects, can all be chosen as fetishes. Usually the fetishist is unmarried, and uses his fetish as an aid to sexual arousal and subsequent masturbation to orgasm; but when the fetishist does marry he is incapable of obtaining erection and subsequent orgasm unless his partner or himself wears or holds the fetish during lovemaking.

Among the fetishists I know are a fur-fetishist—he can only make love satisfactorily if his partner, naked, is swathed in quite costly furs; a white-boot fetishist, who can only get an erection and subsequently obtain orgasm if his partner wears a pair of white—no other color will do—calf-high boots when they make love—a pantie fetishist, who can only make love successfully if he holds a pair of women's panties, as he stimulates a partner; and a homosexual hair-fetishist who can only become sexually aroused and achieve orgasm if his partner has a mass of body hair covering belly and chest.

The fetishist is not only a harmless individual, his fetish is also a harmless preoccupation (except possibly in the case of the pantie fetishist, who is often tempted to steal panties off clotheslines and thereby fall foul of the law, though the married pantie fetishist generally manages to avoid the temptation) and should not really be unacceptable to any partner. For a woman to cooperate should not be at all difficult unless she is unwilling to surrender her prudery and false modesty to expressing her love. Personally I doubt whether a woman who cannot cooperate in all but the most extreme forms of deviation is really sincerely in love with her partner. Like most deviations, fetishism can be treated by psychotherapy, but usually a long course and extensive reeducation is required, and I do not really see the point of it, unless it is a really bizarre fetish which no woman should be required, or expected, to play any part in.

There is one deviation, however, which very often intrudes in a marriage and can have very unfortunate consequences for the relationship. Nevertheless, I know three women who have been able to cope with it, so it shows that it need not be the ogre it is made out to be, or can seem to be, if only the woman loves her husband truly and has the courage to make a mental readjustment which I think is unavoidable.

It sometimes, though fortunately comparatively rarely, happens that a man develops what are known as transvestite tendencies when he has been married some years. A transvestite is a man who has an unconquerable desire to dress in women's clothes. It begins very often with a strong desire to wear women's panties, and as it is fairly easy to do this without much fear of discovery, he yields to temptation. But as time passes, panties alone are not enough to satisfy the desire, and gradually the full wardrobe, plus high-heeled shoes, make-up, and jewelry are essential to meet the transvestite demands.

Now it does not take much imagination to appreciate in what a predicament this places the married man. He cannot resist the impulse to dress in women's clothes, but having provided himself with a wardrobe he lives in constant terror that no matter how well he may hide them, his wife may discover them. In order to satisfy his desire he must dress up when his wife is not at home, and then he is on tenterhooks all the time lest she should return home while he is still dressed up. And what is he to do if the desire comes upon him very strongly when his wife is at home and is unlikely to go out?

It is very difficult for the non-transvestite or those who have not come into contact with transvestites to appreciate why a man should have this compulsion to dress in women's clothes. I won't try to explain it, because it would take us too deeply into the realms of psychiatry and probably leave us no wiser at the end of it. But it must be understood that it is a strong compulsion and is practically impossible to eliminate.

So, what is the woman to do who does discover that she is married to a transvestite? Should she reject it, and with it her husband and her marriage; or should she try to come to terms with it, and so keep her husband and preserve her marriage intact? I think it will depend largely on the strength of her character and on the strength of her love for her husband. One thing that may, I think, help her make her decision is this, that although many homosexuals are transvestites, *not all transvestites are homosexuals*. In fact, if a married man is a transvestite, it is not very likely that he will be a homosexual. His dressing up is really an extreme form of fetishism. If they are accepted by their wives, and their wives are agreeable, they generally prefer to make love while wearing their feminine clothes, and the experience is not only more satisfying for them, but because it is, is a more gratifying experience for their wives.

I know that it is impossible for me ever to be in the position of being married to a transvestite, but all my instincts tell me to urge women who find they are to do their best to accept it. There is much to be lost by rejecting it, and a good deal to be gained by accepting it.

All three women I know who are married to transvestites have told me that when they first made the discovery they felt sick, but that this was quickly succeeded by bewilderment, and it was while they were trying to puzzle out why their husbands were behaving in this peculiar way that it struck them that perhaps it might not be so terrible after all. So they talked to their husbands, questioning and probing, and their husbands, relieved not to be secretive and deceiving, and to have someone to talk to, opened their hearts. Once again it was the old, old axiom of the satisfactory sex relationship: Communicate, communicate, communicate.

Once they were reassured that their husbands still loved them and that their sex lives would not be adversely affected, as one of them said, "I believed that if I pretended it was a game in which I could join, there was no reason why I should not cooperate. T's taste in clothes was terrible, so the first thing we did was to get him a whole new wardrobe. I needn't go into details of how we did it, but he's very slim and we chose lingerie together pretending we were buying it for an aunt slightly larger than me. Outer clothes we bought from a first-class mail-order house, and I did what alterations that were necessary to make them fit decently. I taught him how to make-up properly, and though you may think I'm a little 'sick' by now, he does look like a really attractive woman when he's fully rigged out. We were happy enough before, but now that he is no longer afraid of my finding out, he's a much jollier husband, more lighthearted and carefree. He usually wants to dress up about once a week. Sometimes, though not always, he wants to make love to me while he's dressed up. I've got used to that now, too. But we make love two or three times a week like any ordinary man and woman."

As I said earlier, I appreciate how difficult it must be to be able to adjust to this kind of situation, but given a measure of broadmindedness, courage, and love, it can be done. The only alternative is unhappiness.

It may have struck you that I have not so far mentioned homosexuality as a deviation. This is because I flatly refuse to accept homosexuality as a deviation; in my view, it is just another way of life. This is certainly applicable to the hundred percent homosexual. By the very definition of deviation this must be true, for the total homosexual does not vary the ways by which he obtains his sexual satisfaction any more than the total heterosexual does. I believe that it can apply also to the ambisexual; the man or woman, who is quite happy making love to either sex, for any ambisexual will tell you that the experience of making love to a woman is quite different from the experience of making love to a man, and that the quality of the love felt for the respective partner is also quite different. In my view, the ambisexual is really the only person who can make a genuine claim of being in love with two people simultaneously.

There are some alleged experts who advise homosexuals to marry on the grounds that it will cure them of their homosexuality. The more I learn about homosexuals and homosexuality, the more convinced I become that the other school of thought is right—that homosexuality is incurable, and that, therefore, it is quite indefensible to advise a homosexual to marry and equally indefensible for a homosexual to follow the advice. It is also true that a number of homosexuals marry to protect themselves from the hostility which society on the whole still directs toward them. If they marry they will automatically be accepted as heterosexual by an ignorant public. Marriage from such a motive is equally indefensible.

On the other hand there are men who develop homosexual tendencies after they have married, and it is in cases such as this that the really difficult situations may arise, for not only is there the possibility of discovery by the wife, but the added difficulty of the husband trying to adjust to his new sexual awareness, which can be very confusing. The ambisexual who has made love to both sexes throughout his period of sexual maturity has not this difficulty. He is usually very well adjusted both to his heterosexual and his homosexual status. He is fully aware of the difficulties that may confront his marriage relationship if his homosexual activities are discovered by his wife, and he takes extra pains to be discreet so that she shall not be hurt.

It is difficult to advise the woman how to react to her partner's homosexuality. Some women find homosexuality so disgusting that they feel contaminated. Such women have usually had a strictly moral upbringing in which sex is rarely mentioned. When the woman cannot tolerate even the thought of homosexuality, it is better for the couple to separate. On the other hand, when the woman can accept her husband's other way of life, no matter on what conditions, she has nothing to lose by not rejecting him, provided he can continue to fulfill her sexual needs, or has no objection to her seeking fulfillment with a partner outside marriage. The late developer in homosexuality, who has had several years of heterosexual experience, does not, as a rule, like the born homosexual, find it absolutely impossible to take part in heterosexual lovemaking, and so is able to continue to satisfy his wife's needs. If he is so discreet in his homosexual activities that she can never know when he has been with his boyfriend, she may, fairly easily, teach herself to pretend that the boyfriend does not exist. Should she feel that this is better than breaking up the marriage, in my view, she is quite entitled to come to such an arrangement with her husband. Such arrangements can work well, but in my view there should be an agreement between the couple that if the wife should find another partner with whom she could have a fully rounded relationship, the husband should not stand in her way. Most men in this situation will readily agree to such an arrangement because it will free them to make the most of their own homosexual needs.

As in all cases where there are sexual difficulties of any kind, talking it out is absolutely essential. If the couple can sit down and calmly put forward and then discuss each and each other's point of view, a solution can always be found.

Please, if you are confronted with any problems of the type I have dealt with in this chapter, insist on talking it over. Many a marriage has been saved and has continued to be a happy one merely because the couple were able to discuss what difficulties there were, calmly, honestly, and totally.